P9-CFU-884

$ 9.95

from
PROPOSAL
to PUBLICATION

An Informal Guide
to Writing about
Nursing Research

from
PROPOSAL
to PUBLICATION

An Informal Guide
to Writing about
Nursing Research

Elizabeth M. Tornquist

Editor-in-Residence
School of Nursing
University of North Carolina at Chapel Hill
Chapel Hill, North Carolina

ADDISON-WESLEY PUBLISHING COMPANY

Health Sciences Division, Menlo Park, California
Reading, Massachusetts • Don Mills, Ontario • Wokingham, England
Amsterdam • Sydney • Singapore • Tokyo • Madrid
Bogotá • Santiago • San Juan

For Amy, Joel, Mary, and Mama

Sponsoring Editor: Nancy Evans
Production Supervisor: Anne Friedman
Interior and Cover Designer: Richard Kharibian
Copyeditor: Edith P. Lewis

Library of Congress Cataloging-in-Publication Data

Tornquist, Elizabeth M., 1933–
  From proposal to publication.

  Includes index.
  1. Nursing—Authorship.   2. Nursing—Research.
I. Title.   [DNLM: 1. Writing—nurses' instruction.
WZ 345 T686f]
RT24.T67 1986   808'.06661   86-8009
ISBN 0-201-08012-5

ABCDEFGHIJK—MA—89876

Some of the material in Part Three appeared in a slightly different form in "Strategies for
Publishing Research," published in *Nursing Outlook*, May/June, 1982, and is used with the
permission of the American Journal Nursing Company. Copyrighted material from the
following journals has been used, with permission, to illustrate well written articles
reporting research: *Advances in Nursing Science, American Association of Nephrology Nurses
and Technicians Journal* (now the *American Nephrology Nurses Association Journal*), *The
American Journal of Maternal Child Nursing, American Journal of Nursing, Association of
Operating Room Nurses Journal, The Canadian Journal of Psychiatric Nursing, Cancer
Nursing, Geriatric Nursing, Heart & Lung, The Journal of Continuing Education in Nursing,
Journal of Nurse Midwifery, The Journal of Nursing Administration, Journal of Nursing
Education, Journal of Obstetric, Gynecologic and Neonatal Nursing, Nurse Educator, The
Nurse Practitioner: The American Journal of Primary Care, Nursing Administration
Quarterly, Nursing and Health Care, Nursing Management, Nursing Research, Oncology
Nursing Forum, Pediatric Nursing, Research in Nursing and Health*, and *Western Journal of
Nursing Research*.

Addison-Wesley Publishing Company
Health Sciences Division
2725 Sand Hill Road
Menlo Park, California 94025

Contents

PART FOUR   Adjuncts to Preparing Research
Proposals, Reports, and Articles   185

Preface

This handbook is for nurses who would like help in writing about their research. The suggestions are intended primarily for beginning researchers, but some of them will also be useful to the more seasoned, who may want a review or need the answer to a question. The three main parts of the book provide guides to the three types of writing related to research—the proposal; the thesis, dissertation or research report; and the article reporting research. Some bits of advice are in a concluding section.

I have tried to make each of the main parts reasonably complete and self-contained, without a great deal of repetition; and I have cross-referenced to help fill the gaps. But inevitably, both gaps and overlaps remain. For example, because the literature review for a research proposal is much like that for a thesis or dissertation, I have not discussed the review in any depth in the part on writing a thesis or dissertation; instead I have made only a few brief suggestions for changes from the proposal. So when you write the review for a thesis you may need to refer to the suggestions on writing a proposal. On the other hand, since there are both similarities and differences in the methods section of a proposal and that of the thesis, I have described methods in both places and the descriptions overlap.

The book is meant to be used as a guide when you write. If you read it straight through you will find it repetitious, so I suggest that you read it like a cookbook: look up the recipe you want just before you begin or when you need a reminder about what to do next. I have kept the style informal since this is a practical handbook, not a treatise on writing. I hope you will find it readable and helpful.

Elizabeth M. Tornquist

Acknowledgments

I would like to thank a number of people who have been helpful to me in writing this book. My colleagues Dr. Mary Champagne, Dr. Cynthia Freund, Dr. Sandra Funk, Ruth Ouimette, and Dr. Ingrid Swenson read parts of the manuscript and made many helpful comments. Edith P. Lewis's editorial suggestions greatly improved the manuscript, and Kathy Holladay and Michael Neelon typed it patiently, promptly, and well through innumerable drafts and revisions.

I am indebted to Nancy Evans of Addison-Wesley, who drew me into this exciting project and saw me through it with just the right blend of help and prodding, and to Drs. Virginia and Francis Neelon, who encouraged and supported me throughout the months of writing and rewriting. I am grateful to my friend Joyce Semradek, who first brought me to work with nurses, and to Dean Laurel Archer Copp of the School of Nursing of the University of North Carolina at Chapel Hill, who saw the utility of having an editor on her faculty and has kept me happily working with nurses for a decade.

Finally, I owe a great debt of gratitude to the graduate students I have worked with at the School of Nursing over these years. They have taught me most of what I know about nursing research and have shown me both the problems in writing about the research and the solutions. This is really their book.

PART ONE

Writing a Research Proposal

Chapter 1

The Basic Outline

The purpose of a research proposal is to justify what you plan to do in order to gain approval for it. The proposal must do four things: (1) establish the context for your study and demonstrate a need for it; (2) show that your study will meet the need, using the methods you propose; (3) give assurances that the study will not harm its subjects; and (4) indicate what you will do with the information you collect. If you needed no approval from others, no funds or facilities, no subjects to work on, you would never have to write a formal proposal—you could just decide what you wanted to do, and do it. The need to obtain approval does have a fringe benefit, however, because developing a proposal forces you to think through the project all the way to the end. Thus you can prepare for problems in advance, so that midway through the study you don't find yourself saying, "If only I had seen this coming."

The writer of a research proposal has a great advantage over most other writers: the basic outline already exists. You don't have to invent it, all you have to do is follow it. This basic outline is essentially the same for research projects, theses, and dissertations, no matter how much they may vary in complexity. (For a grant proposal, the organization differs somewhat, but the content remains much the same. See Part Four, pages 202–207, for a brief discussion of the organization of grant proposals.) The basic outline follows. More detailed outlines and descriptions of the various parts of a proposal are given in later chapters.

Proposal Outline

I.   Introduction and review of the literature
  A. The problem needing a solution, the question to be answered, or the theory to be tested
  B. The work already done or prior tests of the theory
  C. Gaps or shortcomings in the work done to date
  D. The purpose of the present study

II. Methods
  A. The design of the study (overview, hypotheses, and research questions)
  B. Setting and sample
  C. Intervention, if applicable
  D. Variables and their measurement
  E. Research procedures

III. Plans for analysis and use
  A. The data expected
  B. Types of analyses planned
  C. Uses of the outcomes
  D. Limitations of the study

This outline enables you to tell others why you will do a study (the introduction and literature review), how you will do it (methods), and to what end (analysis and use). With that logic in mind, it's easier to go about writing.

But much of the work comes before writing begins. To produce a research proposal you need to think, read, and write—in that order, though you also need to write, think, and read; and to read, think, and write. The process goes round and round and back and forth. First you read and think, then you write, and as you write you think more. You also see the flaws in what you have already thought and written, so you go back to thinking. Then you write again, and because writing is discovery, you often find that you have ideas and questions and even information that you didn't know you had. That leads you to new reading and further analyses and thus to new and different writing. So the process goes.

Although writing and thinking cannot really be separated, this handbook is primarily about writing, not about thinking. It assumes you have already thought through most of what you are proposing; the suggestions here are for putting your thoughts in the form of a proposal. Emphasis is on those sections of the proposal that seem to pose writing problems primarily (the literature review, for example), with only passing consideration given to areas in which the problems are mainly thinking problems (plans for analysis, for example). The text follows the basic Proposal Outline on page 4, but you may not write in that order.

In fact, you're quite unlikely to write in that order. For example, the purpose statement is usually the concluding sentence in the literature review, but you cannot write the review until you know what the purpose of your study is; otherwise the review will have no direction. So it's helpful to write out the purpose statement before you begin writing the review, and keep it beside you as a guide to where you're going. (Later you may find that you need to alter the purpose statement, since the very act of writing and thinking about the literature can help you further refine your goals.) Most people find it helpful to write the review of the literature while they are still working out their methods. That saves time and also allows them to check their thinking about methods as they describe others' work. Some people, however, find it easier to write a draft of their methods first and use that as a basis for conceptualizing the literature review. Wherever you begin, save the opening section of your proposal—the introduction—for last.

Chapter 2

Introduction

The introduction to a proposal is an abstract of its first major section—the section I have called "Introduction and Review of the Literature." Whether you need this introduction depends on the complexity of the literature you must review in order to establish a context for the study. Some studies are set squarely upon others, like building blocks; the logic of the literature review is simple and linear. But some literature reviews must pull together research in several apparently unrelated areas to develop a rationale for the study. Here, the argument is not simple but many-branched and intricate.

For example, the early studies of the effectiveness of relaxation in reducing chemotherapy-induced nausea and vomiting had to pull together the literature in a number of areas—problems of side effects of cancer chemotherapy, inadequacy of pharmacological treatment, relation of side effects to stress, and capacity of relaxation to reduce other stress-related problems—to make a case for trying relaxation therapy as a way to reduce nausea and vomiting in cancer patients. In contrast, later studies of the use of relaxation therapy needed mainly to review the earlier studies, pointing both to their encouraging findings and to the methodological shortcomings that made further study necessary, before this therapy could be widely recommended.

If the argument of your literature review is simple and linear, readers probably will not need a separate introduction to your study. You can begin with a description of the problem you intend to solve, the question you will answer, or the theory you intend to test, then review the studies that have already tested solutions to the problem, and conclude with your purpose.

For example, if you plan to do another study of relaxation as a means to reduce nausea and vomiting, you can quickly establish the problem (it's so well known you won't need to say much), then review the reported studies, discuss their shortcomings to establish the need for yet another study, and, finally, indicate how your study will meet that need. Your opening argument might be something like this: "Cancer chemotherapy is effective in an increasing number of cases, but for many patients side effects such as nausea and vomiting are so severe that they make the treatment seem almost worse than the disease. Pharmacological agents are effective in some cases, but not all. Several studies have indicated that relaxation techniques can reduce the nausea and vomiting. . . ." Thus, in only a few short sentences, you give the reader a good idea where you are going.

If, however, you must pull together literature from several areas to establish the rationale for the study, you cannot immediately show readers where you are going. This is often the case when the solution you are testing has been used for other problems but not for the one in which you are interested. Suppose, for example, you want to test the effectiveness of a structured exercise program in improving agility and strength in the elderly. Let's assume that there have been no prior studies of this kind. You must pull together the literature on lack of activity among the elderly, the relation of age and inactivity to strength and agility, the effect of exercise on strength and agility in other age groups where this has been tested, and so on. The complexity is such that no matter what your starting point, readers cannot see where you are headed. They need a road map. In that case, it is best to give a brief overview or abstract of your literature review in a separate introductory section. In other words, present the rationale for the study immediately so that readers can stay with you once you plunge into the literature.

Ideally, this introductory section consists of only a few paragraphs that (1) delineate the problem, the question, or the theory to be tested; (2) discuss in three or four sentences the most relevant work done on the subject; (3) present the need for further work; and (4) give the purpose of the study, with perhaps a sentence or two about its potential usefulness for nursing. Don't label this material "Introduction." The fact that it is introductory in nature will be obvious from its content.

The introduction is relatively easy to write once you have written the literature review. For the opening paragraph on the problem or question or theory, condense the first couple of pages of the review into one paragraph. Look at your purpose statement to help you focus the condensation and ensure a good fit.

To write the two or three paragraphs you need on the research already done on the problem, work from the concluding paragraphs of your literature review — the ones that draw together the closely related work and discuss gaps or shortcomings. You may need to add more details about the methods and findings of the most relevant studies to give readers enough information to follow your thinking, but be brief. Then copy your purpose statement from the conclusion of the review. If it seems appropriate, you can rephrase the purpose or state it more generally than in the literature review.

If you are proposing to test a solution to a problem, you will not need to point out the practical usefulness of your study; that will be obvious. But if you aim to answer a question whose importance for practice is not immediately clear, it is helpful to add a sentence or two making that connection for readers.

Sometimes people go further and include hypotheses or research questions or even discuss methods in the introduction. That is both unnecessary and unwise. Again, remember to think of the introduction only as an opening statement to provide readers a road map for what lies ahead.

Introduction is only a guide for the reader.

Chapter 3

Review of the Literature

Because organizing and writing the literature review can be a very complex operation, the material to follow has been divided into three main sections: (1) organizing the material; (2) writing the review; and (3) specific writing suggestions.

SECTION 1 ORGANIZING THE REVIEW

Research studies differ in the way they are related to the existing body of literature. In this sense your study will probably be one of four major types: (1) a study that tests or extends theory; (2) one that does not test theory but uses a theoretical model as a framework for solving a problem or answering a question; (3) one that has no explicit theoretical framework but simply sets out to answer a question or test a solution to a problem; or (4) one that replicates, directly or indirectly, an earlier study. The type of study determines the organization of the first section of the proposal, the introduction and review of the literature.

Organizing According to Study Type

Testing a Theory.   If your study will attempt to test or extend theory, first describe the theory, then discuss the empirical research already done to test the theory, delineate the work still needing to be done, and conclude with what you plan to do.

Using a Theoretical Model to Solve a Problem or Answer a Question.   A study that does not test theory but uses a theoretical model as a framework for solving a problem or answering a question is organized quite differently. First establish the existence and importance of the problem or question, then discuss the research already done to solve the problem or answer the question. Then— and only then—present the conceptual framework for the proposed solution or answer. Next, discuss any previous use of this framework or model in your problem area, review the flaws or gaps in the research, and conclude with the purpose.

A caution: Sometimes people have the idea that the theoretical framework must always be presented first in the literature review, but they fail to distinguish between testing a theory and using a theoretical model to frame a solution to a problem or answer a question. If you describe the theoretical model first, you present the solution before the problem—a classic case of the cart before the horse. What is likely to happen then is that, having discussed the framework for the solution, you next discuss the problem, and finally, realizing that logically you must move from problem to solution, you end up describing the framework for a solution again. Thus you have cart, horse, and cart again—something like the old pioneer wagons in their circle for the night. You will avoid that illogic if you remember the simple rule that problem always precedes solution.

Studies Without an Explicit Theoretical Framework.   If there is no explicit theoretical framework, there is generally no need for a discussion of theory. Let's say, for example, that you have observed a problem in patient care and you know that some efforts have been made to solve it but with inconclusive results or small samples, so you see a need for more research. You are proposing to test a new solution or treatment. There is no explicit theory behind the treatment you plan, however.

For this kind of study establish the existence of the problem, discuss the work that has been done, tell why more work is needed, then state your purpose. Mention theory only if some of the work that has been done on the problem is in fact theoretical work.

Sometimes people feel they absolutely must discuss theory or provide some kind of theoretical framework for what they do, so they pull out a theory, no matter how remotely related, and toss it into the literature review. That merely confuses matters. Use a theory only if it is helpful to your argument. If you are pressed to provide a theoretical framework when you can find no useful explicit theory, solve the problem by articulating the more general theoretical underpinnings for your study—the assumptions and conceptualizations on which your expectations are based. Don't drag in a peripheral theory.

Replication Studies. Replication studies are important in every field of knowledge, for replication is the basis of science. In nursing, replication studies have particular importance. The nature of patient care research makes it hard to obtain large samples or to select them randomly and control for variables that might confound the findings. Thus it is rare that a study testing an improvement in patient care can be easily generalized. Replication helps to establish the generalizability that methods in the real world often cannot achieve.

Although the emphasis is different, a replication study has the same basic outline as other studies that aim to solve a problem or answer a question. First, describe the problem, emphasizing its importance in order to lay the foundation for studying it again. Next, briefly review the literature leading up to the study you will replicate; then describe that study in detail and conclude by indicating why you will replicate it.

Organizing the Raw Material

You have probably made quite a stack of notes on the literature you have read, and you may also have a stack of photocopied articles reporting studies that are particularly important or closely related to what you plan. How do you fit all that material into a literature review? An outline will help you organize logically and then you cannot fail to write a coherent review; organization is the key to coherence. If your literature review makes a logical argument, any other faults will be easy to deal with.

To begin, decide into which of the preceding four categories of studies your study falls and make a general outline accordingly. For example, suppose the aim of your literature review is to justify a test of the effectiveness of short-term group therapy in reducing depression among elderly nursing home residents. You have a problem—depression in the elderly—and you are proposing to try a solution. You have no explicit theoretical framework. The basic outline for this type of literature review has three parts: (1) the problem, (2) the work done on the problem, and (3) flaws or gaps in the research. The review then concludes with the purpose of your study.

Next, take your note cards and photocopied articles and put them into stacks by subjects. You probably have a stack on depression in general—theories of causation, behavioral manifestations, effects; you may have a stack on psychological problems in the elderly, including depression, and a stack on the elderly in nursing homes; you probably have some notes on the pharmacological treatment of depression, a collection on the effect of various types of therapy for depression, and some cards on the effects of group therapy in particular. Then you have another stack on the use of psychotherapy among the elderly and some articles describing measurement tools to establish levels of depression.

Sometimes people take their stacks of note cards, separate them by subject, summarize what's on the cards, and call that a literature review. It is not. The literature review should pull together relevant research to establish the context for your study, show how you will build on other work, and indicate a need for what you plan to do. A review of other studies, if organized only by subject, cannot develop the context for yours because it will not show the connections between research in different areas or indicate how your plans are based on others' research.

Once you have your note cards in stacks, don't stop there. Let's assume that you have three main headings in your review outline: the problem, work done on the problem, and flaws or gaps in that research. Put the subject piles together under the appropriate headings.

Now, take the stacks of material for each of the three headings and from them make a detailed outline of the points you want to include in that section of the review. If you are one of the many who find outlining very difficult if not impossible, underline the main points on your cards, label them "I's" if related to the problem, "II's" if general background on solutions, and "III's" if closely related work. Then transfer them to a sheet of paper and you have a general outline.

Here's a rational way to arrange your points within each section of the outline. Organize so that you move from known to unknown, from theoretical work to empirical evidence, from general to particular, from peripheral to highly relevant. The more general the material, the less space you should give to it.

Let's use the study of short-term therapy for depression in the elderly as an example again. For your problem section you have material on depression in general and material on depression in the elderly, particularly in nursing homes. You want to move from general to particular, expanding the discussion as you go. So, for the outline, first jot down a few points about depression in general, next make a few more points about depression as a problem in the elderly, and then present as fully as you can the scope of the problem in nursing homes. Thus the closer you get to your problem, the fuller your outline becomes.

Use the same organizing principle for discussing work already done on the problem. You probably have some material on approaches other than therapy that have been tried, and on their lack of success. Since you are not planning to use these approaches, you don't want to deal with the material at length, but you need to include it since this is part of why you have chosen therapy as a means of reducing depression. Because this material is least related to your work, deal with it first.

Next, let's say you have material on the effects of long- and short-term therapy for depression, group therapy, and psychotherapy for the elderly. The peripheral points should be brief, and closely related work should be discussed more fully. For the outline, first note some general points about the effects of therapy on depression. Then, since long-term therapy is not what you plan to study, note its use and list its disadvantages to explain why it is not the treatment of choice—your choice, anyway—for the elderly. Next list the studies of short-term and group therapy, noting all the findings that will make the case for testing short-term group therapy with the elderly.

The final section of your literature review—gaps or shortcomings in the research done to date—is usually the shortest section, since it does not introduce any new work but merely pulls together and discusses the work you have already examined. This is also likely to be the sketchiest section in the outline because these points are difficult to make until you've written a draft of the literature review and can see what needs to be pulled together. You probably won't have many notes; jot down any ideas you have about the overall gaps or flaws in the studies you've listed.

As you outline, give all your notes and articles a number or letter corresponding to their place in the outline, so you don't forget where they fit. When you have completed the outline, check its logic. Is there a clear order to your points within each section? Do the studies listed discuss solutions to your particular problem or offer answers to your question? Do they make a coherent context for your study? Have you noted gaps or flaws in the research? If the outline seems to you reasonably complete and logical, you are ready to write.

SECTION 2 WRITING THE REVIEW

The first paragraph of a literature review, like the first paragraph of anything else, is the hardest to write and the hardest to make right. Your detailed outline can help you begin. Put the points into sentences, expand where necessary, and move thus from outline to paragraph. If you are one of those people who cannot bear outlining, put your stack of materials beside you, put the points in order, and transfer them from notecards to the page. If nothing helps you do the first paragraph, skip it. Take a blank sheet of paper, write "Paragraph 1" at the top, put it aside, then get out another sheet, write "Paragraph 2" at the top and begin there. (Sometimes it's easier to write the first paragraph last.)

Once you start the first draft, it is important to keep going straight through to the end. If there are still holes in your argument, you can make a note in the margin to go back to the library later. Don't go to the library in the middle of writing a draft. It is too tempting to stay there, to say to yourself, "I can't do this literature review, I haven't read enough." Perhaps you haven't, but chances are that you've read enough for a draft — and more.

The contents of the literature review vary according to the type of study. If you're not testing a theory, for example, you obviously don't need a section describing theory. Below are suggestions for writing all the possible parts of a review; select what's useful for you or most appropriate for your study.

Establishing a Problem or Question

First describe the problem or question that your study will attempt to solve. Perhaps the mortality from breast cancer is high, yet women are not doing the simple breast self-examination that would allow early detection and possible cure. Or perhaps nurses are not giving pain medications frequently enough. Or it is not clear whether and under what circumstances nurse practitioners are cost effective.

In describing a problem, present evidence of its importance, citing whatever authorities are needed to establish its broad existence or its severity in the cases in which it does exist. It is also helpful to cite your own clinical experience or observations as evidence of the problem and its importance. If the problem does not appear serious in itself, point out its connection to problems that *are* serious. For example, suppose the problem you will attempt to solve is sleep interruptions in intensive care units. In describing the problem, point out the serious physiological and psychological problems to which lack of sleep is related.

If you are planning to answer a question or series of questions, give the reasons for considering them important. Cite other authors, use your own experience, and draw connections to serious problems just as you would in establishing the importance of a problem.

If you are replicating a study and the original investigator described the problem well, simply summarize that description, indicate that the problem is ongoing, and add any new information on scope or severity. If the original investigator's description was thin, however, you may need to add more details to convince readers that the problem merits further study.

Sometimes you are concerned with a problem or question that is much larger than the particular aspect you'll study. You must sketch the broad outlines before you can narrow the focus, but do it briefly. The larger the problem, the more widely it is recognized, the more that is known about it, then the more difficult it will be to say anything new and interesting on the subject. For example, if you are going to study some small aspect of the care of patients with lung cancer, you may need to begin by reminding the reader that lung cancer is widespread and most frequently fatal, but you do not need to say much more. The people who will read your review are probably familiar with the statistics on its prevalence, and many have experienced or observed its consequences. Don't repeat what your audience already knows unless you need to make sure the audience knows that you know. (You sometimes have to do the latter for thesis or dissertation readers. You must show your background work to let the committee members know that you have searched the literature or to indicate how you developed your reasoning.)

As you write this section on the problem or question, you are likely to find that you have more general information than information specific to your problem or question. That's because you needed to read broadly to establish a context for thinking about your study; now, however, you must let go much of that general information. Although you spent a lot of time reading to gain a background for the study, your readers shouldn't have to do that. The possible exception, again, may be your thesis committee.

For example, suppose you are going to study the effect of relaxation in reducing some stress-related problem. You will begin the literature review by discussing the particular problem you propose to study and providing evidence that it is stress-related. To do so you must have a clear sense of what the stress response is, and that in turn means you have to understand stress theory, which is the background for your study, its conceptual framework. You don't have to explain all of the theory to readers, however; you can count on them to know. A quick reference to stress theory will suffice, and you can move on to discuss the relation of your particular problem to stress.

Similarly, you don't need to write a review of the whole history of a problem if you are going to examine only one of its current manifestations. And you don't need to spend a lot of time explaining why some broad change in health care has occurred when you are planning to study one of its consequences.

You may find it difficult to prune the general information accumulated through your reading on the problem; you've mastered all this material so you want to display it for others. But most proposal readers will prefer brevity and conciseness. Moreover, the article you will eventually write reporting this research can have only a brief introductory literature review, and very little of that will be on the problem. The more you cut now, the less you'll have to trim later.

Describing a Theory to Be Tested

If your study will attempt to test or extend theory, begin the literature review by describing the theory in enough detail so that readers who are unfamiliar with it can understand what is being tested. And if you are testing two competing theories, describe both. If a theory is new or not well known, it is helpful to describe briefly the research that led to its development, but in most cases it is unnecessary to give details on how the theory came about. The synthesis, which is theory, should be the beginning. Any modifications to the theory that have resulted from other tests of it, however, should be described here. For example, if you plan to test a modified version of the theory that stresssful life events are associated with the onset of disease, present the modified version here, not later in the narrative.

Describing the Work Previously Done

Replication Studies.   If yours is a replication study, a lengthy literature review is unnecessary since the context for your work is provided by the study you will replicate. (Be sure to read all the works referred to in the report of that study, however; it's unwise to depend on another's interpretations.) Very briefly summarize the literature leading up to the original study and add any relevant research the investigator missed. Then describe in detail the study you plan to replicate, pointing out the importance of the findings and describing those aspects of the study that stand in the way of its generalizability.

If other studies have been done since that one, discuss their findings here and indicate why yet another study is warranted. If the other studies are critical of the original study's methods, it is particularly important to say why those are still the best methods or indicate why and how they need modification.

Studies Testing Theory. If you are testing a theory the other studies that have tested that theory should be discussed. You should also discuss those studies that shed light on the adequacy of the theory's portrayal of reality, or usefulness for prediction or prescription. Include not only the studies that support the theory but those that question it.

If the theory makes predictions in several areas, it is not necessary to go into detail about research in those areas you are not testing. For example, if your interest is in the psychological aspects of stress theory, you do not need to describe all the physiological tests of the theory. It is helpful, however, to refer at least generally to this other work. Do not describe here those studies that have led to modifications of the theory. They come earlier in the narrative with the description of the theory itself, for the theory you are testing is the theory with whatever changes have already come about in it.

Studies to Solve a Problem or Answer a Question. If you are planning to test a solution to a problem or answer a question, describe the work already done on the problem or question, moving from theoretical discussions to empirical research. But don't give the two types of work separate headings—"Theoretical Framework" and "Review of the Literature"—as if theory were not part of the literature.

When you discuss other studies, move from peripheral to the more relevant, paying particular attention to studies whose approach to the problem was similar to the approach you plan. There is no need to go into detail about studies not closely related to your plans; for those you need only mention findings. Lump similar findings together into a general statement such as: "There is evidence that a planned teaching program is more effective than incidental instruction." Don't mention all the articles that provide the evidence, just cite them. Sometimes people say, "There is evidence that X affects Y," and then they tell readers that John Doe found X affected Y, and Sara Sloe found X affected Y, and Mary Mahoe found X affected Y, and so on ad nauseum. Don't do that. Never make the same point twice (or more than twice!) just to display your knowledge of the literature. Make it once and give as many references as you like.

If a series of studies have produced overlapping but differing results, or have approached the question from slightly different angles, introduce them with a sentence that tells readers they are related, and then discuss them together. For example, you might begin by saying, "There is evidence that X is associated with Y"; then mention each study, calling attention to the differences and inconsistencies in their findings about the relationship between X and Y.

The closer a reviewed study is to what you plan, the more you must describe its methods. What are the crucial things to say? The numbers studied, diagnosis, intervention, reason for the intervention, or the question explored and why. If the findings are important for your study, describe also the measurement techniques that were used and the type of sample selection. Depending on what you are proposing, you may even need to give information on the ages or economic conditions of the people in the previous study or the location of the research.

For example, if prior studies on parents' views of sex education in schools have all been done in northern urban areas and you plan to study a rural southern population, then it is crucial to mention where the other studies were done. Or if you plan to explore changes in taste among children receiving cancer chemotherapy and all the earlier studies were on adults, you need to make that age distinction clear. In most other cases, it's pointless to give this kind of information.

To decide, ask yourself what readers need to know in order to understand the shortcomings or gaps in the previous research (e.g., no studies of rural southern parents, no studies of children's taste changes while undergoing chemotherapy). Even when other studies are quite close to your own, you should not summarize them. The aim is to give readers just enough information to show why others' findings are useful to build on but not yet acceptable as definitive.

Never ignore studies that tend to argue against your plans or raise questions you cannot answer. To deal with material that conflicts with your views or raises questions about your potential for success, remember that you have looked at the material and decided that its argument was not compelling; otherwise you would not be planning this particular study. The task now is to articulate your reasoning so that readers will make the same decision. For example, why not use pharmacological treatment for depression in the elderly instead of the more expensive and time-consuming therapy you are planning? Clearly you think that the drugs have some shortcomings and that your proposed therapy has advantages that make it worth a try. To convince readers, you need to show them your reasoning.

Where do you put this kind of material? It's hard to say. Logically, studies that argue against what you plan should be described near the end of the literature review since your answer to them is to point out the flaws in their argument, and flaws in the research to date are best presented in your concluding paragraphs. But if there are other studies whose approach is closer to yours, discuss these troublesome studies earlier in the review. You should conclude with a discussion of the studies on which you are directly building.

Unfortunately, that is only one of several tough decisions about placement you're likely to face. No matter how clearly and completely you outline the review, there will be hard choices when you begin to write, because your argument can advance in different ways. For example, some of the work already done on the problem may appear either peripherally or closely related to your proposed study, depending on how you view it. Thus, your conceptualization will determine your placement of the material.

Let's use the study of short-term therapy for depression in the elderly as an illustration. Where should you put material on psychotherapy for the elderly? That depends on how you think of it. If you view psychotherapy for both young and old as a general topic and therapy for depression as more specific to your study, you will first briefly discuss the research on psychotherapy for the elderly, then move to a fuller discussion of therapy for depression. On the other hand, if you consider therapy for depression in people of all ages to be the general topic and psychotherapy for the elderly as more closely related to your study, you'll reverse the order and alter the emphasis.

In order to decide where to put material, ask yourself: What is the logic of my argument? Sometimes you can't answer that question satisfactorily until you have written a first draft and can look at its organization. Then you may find you need to move things around, try them in a couple of places, and see where they fit best. It's particularly difficult to get the organization right the first time when there's little directly related work and you must pull together research in several peripheral areas. Then you will need to play with the arrangement to get the best flow.

Describing a Theoretical Model

If you are using a theory or theories as a basis for proposing a new solution or answer to a problem, describe this theoretical model after reviewing other work already done on the problem. Then discuss the research that has been done to establish the usefulness of the theoretical model. Often you can simply show that this model has worked in some other area and say why you think it will also work here. But you may need to provide evidence that other approaches are less likely to succeed. If the model has worked only in part, tell how you are modifying it to make it more effective. Or indicate how some theory or set of theories provides the basis for your development of a new model. If two competing theories might be useful to you in conceptualizing a solution, describe both.

Describing Gaps and Shortcomings in Previous Work

The section pulling together the work done to date and indicating why more work needs to be done is the most important part of your literature review, since it provides justification for your study. If you are testing a theory that has already been tested, say why it needs to be tested again. Is it because you suspect the previous test to have been inadequate, providing the wrong answers? Is it because the test needs confirmation? Is it because a part of the theory has not been tested at all? Explain the shortcomings in the work already done and say what has not yet been done.

Similarly, if you are using a theoretical model that has already been used in the area of your study, then there must be some shortcomings in the studies that used it, or there would be no need for your study. Point to the flaws in the research to date. Did the solution not work because it was an inadequate test? Did the solution work but on such a small sample that generalization is not warranted? Explain why more work is needed.

If you are answering a question or testing a solution, it is not difficult to show a need for more research if very little work has been done in that area. But if other investigators have already reported a solution to the problem or an answer to the question, you must explain why still more study is warranted. It's particularly important to note other studies' shortcomings as preparation for your purpose. You want to avoid giving readers the impression that your study has already been done.

If there have been only a few studies in your area, describe their shortcomings and the consequences of these at the end of your literature review. But if there are more than a few studies to discuss, mention the aspects of each particular study that constitute limitations as soon as you present the study in your review. Then in the concluding paragraphs, pull the major studies together and, in a summarizing way, discuss their shortcomings and the gaps they leave, or remind readers of the confusing or conflicting data that show the question you're interested in remains essentially unanswered.

This arrangement makes it easier for readers to follow your reasoning. If you explain the problems as you go, readers can probably remember them, and your concluding discussion of shortcomings will make sense. If you don't explain along the way, readers may have trouble figuring out which shortcoming goes with which study and will have to go back and reread to follow what you're saying. You always want to spare readers that kind of extra work. In the final paragraphs you may still have to remind readers of the shortcomings mentioned earlier, but repeat as little as possible. The fewer the studies and the closer they are to the end of the review, the less you need to repeat.

Sometimes it's hard to decide what to do about the shortcomings of particular studies until you have written a draft of the literature review and can look at it to see how much you are expecting readers to hold in mind. If you're not sure which way to go, it's a good idea to give the information as you write. It's easier to go back and cut out unnecessary details than to go back and put in essentials.

Wherever you put things and however you organize, the parts of the literature review should flow together smoothly to establish the context for your study, to show how the study will build on what has already been done, and to indicate how you will take the work further.

Concluding the Literature Review

There are two ways to conclude the literature review. You can end with a purpose statement: for example, "This study will explore the relation between recent life change events and depression in the elderly." (See pages 34–35 for a discussion of purpose statements.) Then you'll begin your "Methods" section with a brief overview of the study, followed by hypotheses or research questions.

Or you can turn your purpose statement at the end of the literature review into a one- or two-sentence overview of your study plans and conclude the review with hypotheses or research questions. In that case, begin the "Methods" section with "Setting and Sample."

Both variants have advantages and disadvantages. The purpose statement makes a nice, neat conclusion to the review of the literature. And the overview that opens the "Methods" section provides a clear introduction to the details that follow. Inevitably, however, there's considerable overlap between the purpose statement and overview, and it may seem repetitious to readers.

The second version avoids that overlap. But if you label, explain, or make a schematic representation of your study design, you must do that before stating hypotheses. It looks peculiar to put your design — so obviously a matter of method — in a section that is not called "Methods" but "Review of the Literature." Also, with this version the "Methods" section begins abruptly.

To decide which version to use, follow your own preference if you have one, your committee's preference if you have a committee, or the preference of journals for which you'll eventually be aiming. (Pointing the proposal in the direction of a publishable article saves both energy and pain later on.)

A research proposal should conclude with a section entitled "Plans for Analysis and Use," which describes intended analyses and potential usefulness of the information you will collect. You may also want to add one or two sentences about these uses at the end of the literature review. It is especially helpful to articulate here the usefulness of the study for nursing if the study is descriptive or correlational and its relation to practice is not immediately clear.

Suppose, for example, you intend to collect data on what mothers of cleft-palate infants know about the care of these infants and the complications that may occur. You might want to tell readers now that this information can be useful to nurses in designing teaching programs and materials that will provide mothers the information they need to help them avoid complications.

If the study includes an intervention, it is rarely necessary to point to intended uses here; they are more or less self-evident. A good rule of thumb is this: The further the research from an obvious practice problem or need, the more important it is to let readers know right away why the study will be useful or what its relation is to some need or problem in nursing.

If your literature review winds up with a purpose statement, follow this with a description of uses. If the review concludes with an overview of the study and hypotheses, however, it is better to work the uses into the overview or put them between the overview and hypotheses. Do not put them after the hypotheses, for that breaks the flow of the proposal's logic; you should always go straight from hypotheses to setting and sample. If it is too difficult to work in the uses when you have hypotheses, it may be best to conclude the literature review with purpose and uses, and save the overview and hypotheses for the beginning of "Methods."

SECTION 3 SPECIFIC WRITING SUGGESTIONS

Making General Points

There are a number of useful constructions for making a general point without going into particular studies.

> It is widely recognized that. . ., *or*
> X is widely recognized (or acknowledged)
>
> It has been well documented that. . ., *or*
> X has been well documented.
>
> It is well known that. . . .

You may or may not need a reference citation for these general points. (See pages 189–191 for a discussion of reference systems. The American Psychological Association [APA] format, used throughout this book, is generally preferred.) If you have more than a very few sentences not requiring a reference to particular authors, however, you are probably spending too much time on the background for your study and may be saying the same thing over and over.

Discussing Several Studies Together

To introduce a summary discussion of other studies there are several variants of the topic sentence, "X affects Y" or "X is better than Y."

> There is considerable evidence that X affects Y. Smith (date), for example, found that. . . .
>
> Several authors (investigators, researchers) have found that X is better than Y. Locke (date) found. . . .

> According to Wilson (date), Pearson (date), Jones (date), and Zollicopher (date), X is better (more effective, efficient, etc.) than Y. Duffy looked at X and Y in . . . .

> According to several authors (Pierce, date; Oates, date; Jones, date; McGovern, date), X affects Y.

> The studies of Donaldson (date) and Cates (date) indicate that X is better than Y. Graham (date) and Storey (date) found that X affects Y.

For all such text references, of course, the complete bibliographic data for the book or article cited must be given in the reference or bibliography section.

Never introduce a discussion of other studies by saying, "A review of the literature revealed that X is better than Y." This is redundant. What you're reporting in this section *is* your review of the literature.

Similarly, never say, "Only two studies of X were found in the literature." Say, "Only two studies of X have been reported," or be less specific: "Only a few studies of X have been reported." When researchers say, "This review revealed only two studies of X," or "Only two studies of X appeared in the literature," or some other version of that statement, they're hoping to convey that they tried to find everything, but maybe they missed a study or two. Don't bother saying it. Readers assume you have made a thorough search of the literature; if by chance they know of a study you did not find, telling them you tried to locate everything will not spare you their irritation.

To condense a lot of related findings into one sentence, this construction is helpful:

> X has had favorable (or unfavorable) outcomes, including A, B, C, and D.

In real language you might write, "These forms of parental inclusion in planning sex education in the schools have had favorable outcomes, including lowered anxiety about the courses (Heart, 1980), fewer negative feelings (Caudle, 1982), enhanced parent-child communication (Holladay, 1983), and greater parental interest in the schools (Miles, 1985)."

Describing Particular Studies in Detail

Introduce a study you plan to discuss in detail with a sentence that gives the main findings together with those aspects of methods (such as sample size) that establish the credibility of the findings. Don't make a long introduction to the study; get to the point quickly. Suppose, for example, you are going to discuss a study that found most children injured in car accidents were not wearing seat belts or other forms of child restraints. You can begin in any one of several ways.

> Jones (date) found that only 3 of 89 children under six who had been injured in car accidents were using restraints.

> Among 89 children under six who had been injured in car accidents, Jones found only 3 were wearing restraints (date).

> Jones (date) examined 89 children under six who had been injured in car accidents; only 3 had used restraints.

> In a study of children under six who had been injured in car accidents, Jones found that only 3 of 89 had been in restraints (date).

Do not split the information into two sentences like this: "Jones examined 89 children under six who had been injured in car accidents. He found only 3 were using restraints." That slows progress and irritates readers, because they have to read a sentence whose importance is not clear until the next sentence.

Often the first sentence, if it does not come to the point, has a meaningless predicate or conclusion, as in the example below:

> Comparing 25 mother–child pairs who had spent hours together immediately after birth with those who had had only brief contact, the authors *found differences*. At three, six, and nine months the bonded babies had gained more weight.

The two sentences can be combined and the meaningless predicate omitted, thus:

> Comparing 25 mother–child pairs who had spent hours together immediately after birth with those who had had only brief contact,

the authors found that the bonded babies had gained more weight at three, six, and nine months.

Combining facts is sometimes difficult, and you may have to try several constructions before getting a good one. For example, look at this collection of data.

Fifteen subjects were studied by Jones to determine taste changes. His sample consisted of five normal controls, five patients with metastasized cancer and five patients post-thoracotomy for malignancy. Although the threshold for bitterness was slightly lower in those with disseminated cancer, the difference was not significant.

It's tough to get all that into one sentence, even if you cut out the vague opening. Here's one way:

Testing five normal controls, five patients with metastasized cancer, and five patients post-thoracotomy for malignancy, Jones found that the only taste change was a slightly lower threshold for bitterness among those with metastasized cancer, and this difference was not significant.

If you cannot get the whole point in one sentence, give the sample size or other important aspects of methods along with the main findings first; then in a second sentence give more detail about specific outcomes. Or give the main findings first and in the next sentence discuss methods. Depending on their importance for your study, both the findings and the methods can usually be summarized in a few sentences. Then mention the methodological shortcomings; if the author concludes there is a need for the kind of research you plan, note that too.

When you describe other studies and their conclusions, don't quote; paraphrase. To quote someone's words is to call special attention to them; this is justifiable only if the words are so extraordinary as to add to the sense by their strength, beauty, conciseness, or all three. Occasionally you find a sentence that you really want to quote. Then do so. Usually, however, people quote because they are too lazy or fearful to paraphrase. And that causes more problems than it solves since a quote rarely fits into the flow of your own argument. You either have an awkward intrusion or you have to write more words around the quote to make it fit in.

Referring to Authors

When you report another's findings, you can name the author in the text or simply mention the study, citing the author in parentheses. You can also introduce the information with a statement like "It has been found (or shown) that . . . ," or turn the finding into a conclusion or general statement.

> Jones (date) found that in the 15 professions he studied, job satisfaction was correlated with occupational prestige.
>
> A study conducted among members of 15 professions found that the greater the occupational prestige, the greater the job satisfaction (reference).
>
> It has been shown that job satisfaction is related to occupational prestige (reference).
>
> The greater the occupational prestige, the greater the job satisfaction (reference).

When you mention an author in the text, give only the last name; omit titles and don't say, "Freud, the noted psychiatrist . . . ." Those who are reading your material are probably as well informed about authorities as you are. If you suspect readers are not informed, tell them gently with a phrase like this: "Smith, in her many years of work with disturbed children, found . . . ."

Do not include the name of the article or book you are discussing; just give the author's name (and in parentheses the date of publication, if you use APA style, or a number for the reference at the end of the sentence if you use another system). There are only rare exceptions to this rule. Before you give the title of a work, ask yourself why readers need to have it in the narrative when they can easily find it in the reference list. Unless you can give yourself a good reason for singling out this work, don't.

When you refer to a study in the text and give only the author's name in a parenthetical reference citation, you must name the author if you then refer to this person in the text. You cannot use a pronoun because a reference citation in parentheses is not part of the narrative and thus will not function as an antecedent for the pronoun.

Similarly, if you make a general statement such as: "The elderly are characterized by stooped posture (Jones, 1980)," you cannot then say in the next sentence, or two sentences later, "Other studies have found similar results." This is because you have mentioned no study in the narrative to serve as a referent for the word "other."

To avoid this kind of problem, either make every statement about a particular study general and give a reference at the end of the discussion, or refer to the author in your first sentence about the study so you can safely use the pronoun for further comments.

Getting the Right Verb Tense

Verb tenses are often a problem. Every good grammar book will tell you to make your tenses consistent, and you may still remember teachers saying not to shift tenses. But there are many choices of tenses, and shifting is sometimes right, sometimes not. So much depends on your precise meaning that it is hard to make general rules about what's consistent, what's right, and what's an unjustifiable shift.

Generally you use the past tense to report others' findings.

> Smith and Kean (date) found that cancer patients did not generally suffer serious body image problems as a result of hair loss following chemotherapy.

Although others' findings are presented in the past tense, their conclusions or suggestions may be stated in the present, especially when you want to indicate that a conclusion remains valid or to emphasize its importance.

> Chadwick and Griffin (date) concluded that body image is not a serious problem for cancer patients with alopecia if they have supportive relationships with family and with physicians.

Always use the present tense to make a general statement about continuing reality.

The incidence of lung cancer among women is increasing.

And use the present tense for statements that are widely agreed on.

It is widely acknowledged that patient teaching is an important fac-
tor in compliance.

The present perfect tense can be used to shift gracefully from
past to present and back again. Look at the verbs in this paragraph
for an example.

The role of patient characteristics in compliance is unclear. Several
authors have explored associations between compliance and patient
characteristics thought to be important. Evans found that poor people were less likely to comply with diet instructions than middle-class
people. Smith, however, found no association between compliance
and socioeconomic status. Other authors have concluded that patient
characteristics are less important than the provider-patient
relationship.

Sometimes you use different tenses to indicate a sequence of
events. For example, to indicate that at some past time repeated
vomiting preceded anticipatory nausea, you would use the past
perfect tense with the past tense.

Jones (date) found that people who had vomited repeatedly after
chemotherapy sometimes experienced anticipatory nausea when
awaiting a treatment.

Sometimes the sequence of events is not so clear or so important,
and you can use the past with the past instead of using the past
perfect.

Price found that patients who lost their hair suffered few problems
with body image.

One way to decide when you should use what tense is to read
the sentence aloud. If it sounds right, it probably is right, for we
tend to speak more naturally and correctly than we write. If you
are still unsure, it's wise to consult a handbook on writing. Johnson's *The Handbook of Good English* has useful hints for getting

verb tenses right and is a good general reference for many other tricky problems. Strunk and White's *The Elements of Style* is equally useful on verbs and other basic points. And most college English handbooks will help you.

Wording

Never write "research concluded" or "these sources think" or "several studies said." You can get away with saying "a study found," but just barely. Only people—authors, investigators, or writers—think, say, find, and conclude.

When you want to point out that someone's research supports a particular view or position, say it just that way. Don't say that the research "supports" a finding or "supports" that something is true. A study can support a position, an argument, a conclusion, or one author can concur with another's view; facts and findings, however, cannot be supported, they can only be confirmed. They can also argue against a position, as can an author. Keep in mind these distinctions.

Never say "prove." That word should be saved for the geometricians. The authors you cite may have found or demonstrated something, or they may have ascertained or determined something. Or, in a slightly less positive way, their studies may indicate or suggest something, or the authors may conclude something. But none of them has proved anything.

In describing what other studies have achieved, try to be as precise as possible and choose words to convey slight variations in meaning. For example, the word "discover" has a little more surprise in it than "find," so you may want to save it for the serendipitous or the disappointing and use "find" for the expected.

"Demonstrate" and "show" have about the same meaning but because "demonstrate" is a bigger word, it has an air of greater certainty and formality about it. "Show" is more modest.

"Ascertain" and "determine" overlap; but "ascertain" means to find out for certain or find the truth. To "determine" is more to settle the question.

To "identify" is to establish the identity of or determine the type. It is not a synonym for "show," "ascertain," "determine," or "find." You might write, "He identified three types of responses," but not, "He identified that patients had three types of responses." Above all, never say "identify" when you mean "define."

Be careful about singulars and plurals when using Latin or Latin-derived words—for instance, criterion/criteria, phenomenon/phenomena, datum/data.

Avoid the word "state" when you mean "say." "State" implies a systematic declaration or a degree of positiveness well beyond "say." Witnesses in the courtroom state, but most other people say things. Occasionally an author states the case for something, but usually authors will only say, and so should you.

A conclusion is a general statement of a situation, usually based on findings. In contrast, a finding is particular. If the findings are strong, their author may have concluded something; if the findings are tentative, use the word "suggest" or "indicate."

Don't use "propose" when you mean "suggest." To "propose" is to put forth something for consideration, as a goal or purpose, or as a theoretical proposition. "Suggest" means to imply or to lead logically to an idea or conclusion. You can use "suggest" to mean "propose," but not the reverse. For example, you might write, "She proposed (or suggested) a study on the effect of primary nursing on patient anxiety," but you could not say, "She proposed that the patient's vomiting resulted from anxiety."

Transitions

Whenever you bring new material into the literature review, make its connection to your argument immediately clear. Otherwise, the reader will think it's a digression and wonder what happened to the main train of thought.

Transitions help tie the sentences and paragraphs together and show readers your logic. They are like road signs, clues to where you're heading. Most grammar books contain lists of common transitional words to indicate addition, cause and effect, comparison, contrast, concession, or to point to examples, time relations, and summaries. It might be helpful to keep such a list beside you as you write.

However, be careful not to tie things together too soon. When you have completed a first draft, you may find that you need to shift sentences and paragraphs around to make your argument logical and coherent. If you have glued the sentences and paragraphs together with transitions, it's harder to unstick them. You may want to aim first at getting the organization right and only then worry about transitions.

Writing the Purpose Statement

If your study is descriptive, you will write the purpose statement that concludes the literature review this way: "The purpose of this study is to explore or discover X or Y or Z (or all of them)." For example, your purpose might be to "discover what families of patients in intensive care need from staff."

If you are looking for correlations, you will say, "The purpose of this study is to ascertain whether X is related to Y (or to Y and Z, etc.)." Or, in real world language, "The purpose of this study is to ascertain whether alcohol abuse by nurses is associated with burn-out syndrome."

If you are predicting a particular type of relation, you will write, "The purpose of this study is to determine whether X increases (or decreases) as Y increases (decreases)." In the language of your study, "The purpose is to determine whether the level of reported pain in patients with bony metastases increases with the level of anxiety."

If the study will include a treatment or intervention, you should say, "The purpose of this study is to determine the effect of X on Y." There are many variants of this statement. You may want to determine whether X will cause Y, improve Y, reduce Y, or alter Y in some other way, or alter both Y and Z, or alter Y without affecting Z, and so on.

You may want to state the purpose more strongly. Suppose, for example, you fully expect a structured exercise program to improve strength and agility in the elderly. You will say, "The purpose of this study is to determine the effectiveness of X (exercise) in improving Y and Z (strength and agility in the elderly)." That statement makes your expectations clear.

Your aims may be more complex, but the basic formulas for stating a purpose are the same. If you cannot fit your purpose statement into one of the formulas, or variants of the formulas, you may need to clarify or simplify your purpose.

Once you have a clear purpose statement, check it against the description of the problem or question or theory in the opening paragraph of the literature review. Do they fit together? Does the purpose statement propose a way to solve the problem, suggest that you will try to answer the question you have raised, or tell the reader that you will test a proposition you've described? If so, you are ready to move on to "Methods."

References

American Psychological Association. (1983). *Publication manual* (3rd ed.). Washington, DC.

Johnson, E. D. (1982). *The handbook of good English*. New York: Facts on File Publications.

Strunk, W., Jr., & White, E. B. (1979). *The elements of style* (3rd ed.). New York: Macmillan.

Chapter **4**

Methods Section for Research Proposals

While the review of the literature must persuade readers that the study you plan is worth doing, the "Methods" section must convince them that the study is feasible. The contents and organization of this section depend on the kind of study being undertaken, so, like the preceding chapter, this one will be divided into two sections. The first presents outlines for various designs, and the second, the individual parts of "Methods." The latter include the overview, hypotheses, research questions, definitions, setting and sample, intervention, data collection instruments, pilot study, and procedure.

SECTION 1 OUTLINES FOR VARIOUS DESIGNS

Quantitative Studies Without an Intervention

Quantitative studies without an intervention may vary considerably in design, but they all follow much the same outline. There are three major types.

1. You plan to collect information about some particular characteristics (variables) of a sample or situation, but you are not predicting what you'll find. You may, for example, plan to collect data on pain, depression, anxiety, body image, and coping strategies in a sample of recovering burn patients.

2. You want to find out whether particular factors or variables in the sample or situation are associated, but you have no basis for predicting these associations. Perhaps, for example, you want to see whether age, race, socioeconomic status, marital status, and parity are associated with use of various types of contraceptives, but you are not predicting these associations.

3. You are predicting associations between variables—for instance, that lifestyle habits will be found to be healthier among those of high socioeconomic status than among the poor.

In all three types of studies the outline is the same except that in the first two you have research questions and in the third you have hypotheses. Here's what the "Methods" section should contain for these three types of study.

Methods

A. The design of the study
 1. Overview of what is planned
 2. Hypotheses or research questions

B. Setting and sample
 1. Characteristics of the setting, if applicable
 2. The source of your sample
 3. Criteria for selecting the sample
 4. Planned sample size

C. Data collection
 1. Variables to be described or measured
 2. Means of collecting the information
  a. Physiological measures, if applicable
  b. Scheduled observations, if applicable
  c. Questionnaires or interviews, if applicable
   For a, b, and c, wherever applicable and available,

          (1) description of the instrument, method of use, and method of scoring
          (2) data on validity and reliability collected by other investigators
          (3) information on pilot testing
          (4) information on interrater reliability
       d. Collection of demographic data, if not included in c above

  D. Procedure for conducting the study
     1. Means of gaining access to the sample
     2. Measures to be taken to protect the rights of human subjects
     3. The data collection process for each participant

Secondary Data Analyses

A study based on an existing data set is not so different from other quantitative studies except that you are not collecting data yourself and thus your "Methods" section is less important than the section called "Plans for Analysis and Use." The outline for the "Methods" section for this type of study looks like this.

Methods

  A. Design of the study
     1. Overview of what is planned, and the variables of interest
     2. Hypotheses or research questions

  B. Description of the data
     1. Source of the data
       a. Population sampled and method of sampling
       b. Data collected and method(s) of collection
     2. Description of the data of interest for the present study

3. Usefulness of the data for measuring the variables of interest in the present study

Studies That Include an Intervention

If you plan to institute a treatment or change an arrangement and then measure the effects of the intervention, the outline of the "Methods" section is somewhat more complex. The outline, however, will be approximately the same whether your study is to be pre-experimental, quasi-experimental, or experimental. The outline is also essentially the same even if your study is designed to evaluate someone else's intervention or program, or is assessing a small treatment that is part of a larger program or study. Here's what the "Methods" section should contain.

Methods

A. Design of the study
   1. Overview of what is planned
   2. Narrative and schematic description of the design, with variables labelled or identified
   3. Hypotheses to be tested and any additional research questions

B. Setting and sample
   1. Characteristics of the setting
   2. Criteria for selecting the sample
   3. Planned sample size
   4. Method of dividing the sample into groups, if applicable (in a time-series design, times at which measurements will be taken)

C. The intervention
   1. Description of the standard program (protocol) for the treatment group(s), or the change to be made, or the ongoing program to be evaluated

    2. The development of the intervention, including any pilot testing

    3. Plans for an intervention with the comparison group, if applicable

D. Data collection

    1. The variables to be observed in order to measure the effects of the intervention

    2. The means of observing the variables

       a. Physiological measures, if applicable

       b. Scheduled observations, if applicable

       c. Questionnaires or interviews, if applicable

       for a, b, and c, wherever applicable and available,

         (1) Description of the tool, method of use, and method of scoring

         (2) Data on validity and reliability from other investigators

         (3) Pilot testing

         (4) Information on interrater reliability

       d. Collection of demographic data, if not included in c above

E. Procedure for conducting the study

    1. Means of gaining access to the sample

    2. Measures to be taken to protect the rights of human subjects

    3. The process each person in the experimental group will go through

    4. The process each member of any comparison group will go through (if this is a time-series design, the order of #3 and #4 may be reversed)

Qualitative Research

Field Studies. The outline for field studies resembles that for quantitative studies without an intervention, though with some modifications. For example, if you plan to observe a situation or part of a population in order to discover its important characteristics, you may not have clearly formulated research questions and you certainly will not have hypotheses. Your plans for sampling may develop only as you go, and you may not even decide exactly how you'll collect data until you get into the situation. Here's a general outline (though the details may be uncertain) for such a study.

Methods

A. Design of the study
   1. Overview of what is planned
   2. Research questions, if to be explicitly stated

B. Setting and sample
   1. The setting for the study
   2. Method of sampling the population under study, if formulated

C. Data collection plans
   1. Participant observations, if applicable
   2. Nonparticipant observations, if applicable
   3. Interviews or questionnaires, if applicable
   4. Document analysis, if applicable

D. Procedures for recording data
   1. Taping
   2. Field notes

Historical Research.   The plans for historical investigations may be even vaguer than for field studies because there's so little you can say ahead of time. Here's a general outline. (Note: people often disagree about the proper labels for research designs. The outline below refers not to retrospective quantitative studies but to explorations of the past.)

Methods

A. Design of the study
   1. Overview of what is planned
   2. Research questions, if to be explicitly stated

B. Data collection plans
   1. Documents to be examined
   2. Persons to be interviewed
   3. Interview schedule

SECTION 2 COMPONENT PARTS OF METHODS

The Overview

The overview is a one- or two-sentence description — almost a skeletal abstract — of the study methods. It gives readers a sense of how you plan to achieve your purpose and provides them with a framework on which to hang the details of what you're planning to do. Thus, the overview functions like a tour map.

If your literature review ended with a purpose statement, begin the "Methods" section with the overview. But if the review concluded with an overview and with your hypotheses or research questions, you don't need to repeat any of them. You can begin "Methods" with a description of the setting and sample.

For a study that does not include an intervention you might write the overview this way:

> In order to discover what patients find stressful about the cardiac care unit, a sample of patients recently transferred from the CCU will be interviewed about their impressions of the unit, using a questionnaire developed by the investigator.

Thus, in one sentence you tell what you will do, when, to whom, in order to find out what. The formula sentence, which could be used for any similar study design, is this:

> In order to gain information on X, a group A will be questioned at time B using means C.

If your purpose is more complex — suppose you intend to seek information on several variables and look at the associations between them — you may need two sentences, such as these:

> In order to discover whether terminally ill patients and their families prefer the dying patient to remain in the hospital or at home, and to find out the reasons for their preferences, a sample of hospitalized terminally ill patients and families will be interviewed about these preferences, using a questionnaire developed by the investigator. Data on diagnoses and patient characteristics will be collected to determine whether these are related to preference for home or hospital care.

These sentences make clear what information you are seeking, what design you will use, who will make up your sample, how you will collect data, and what associations you will explore. Then go on to the details.

For a study that includes a treatment or intervention whose effects will be tested by comparing some outcome in an experimental group with the outcome in a control group, you might write:

> To determine whether relaxation reduces nausea and vomiting in cancer patients receiving chemotherapy, an experimental group will be taught progressive relaxation before receiving therapy, and the frequency and severity of nausea and vomiting in this group will then be compared to nausea and vomiting in a control group who receive no relaxation training.

Here is the basic overview formula for this type of study:

> To test the effectiveness of X in altering Y, an experimental group A will receive X, and the Y in this group will be compared to Y in a control group B who do not receive X.

If you plan to compare the effectiveness of two interventions, for example, routine administration of pain medications versus PRN medications, the overview will be similar.

> To determine whether routinely administered pain medications are more effective than PRN medications in controlling postoperative pain, patients in the surgical ICU will be randomly assigned to a group receiving routine medication or a group receiving PRN medi-

cations, and the reported pain levels within the two groups will be compared.

If you have no comparison group but will compare the experimental group to itself before and after treatment, the overview is like this:

> To determine the effectiveness of relaxation in reducing chronic pain, a group of patients experiencing chronic back pain will be asked to report pain levels before receiving relaxation training and after practicing the technique for six weeks.

The overview should mention all the major variables you plan to observe; this may require two sentences. In the study of the effects of relaxation in reducing nausea and vomiting, for example, you might want to look at both antiemetics received and level of anxiety, so you might write:

> This study will examine the effectiveness of relaxation in reducing nausea and vomiting in cancer patients receiving chemotherapy. An experimental group will be taught progressive relaxation before receiving therapy, and the frequency and severity of nausea and vomiting in this group, as well as antiemetics received and anxiety level before and after therapy, will be compared to a control group who receive no training in relaxation.

As these models show, one of the functions of the overview is to provide a narrative description of your design. In most cases it is not also necessary to label the design; a reader should be able to name it on the basis of what you've written. If you're not sure whether you have provided the appropriate information in your overview, read your description to one or two colleagues and ask them to name the design. If they can't, something may be wrong with the overview, or this may be one of those rare cases in which a label is required. (Sometimes thesis and dissertation committees require you to label the design, not because they need the information, but for evidence that you know what you're doing.)

The most frequent problem is that the overview leaves out essential information while saying other things twice. For example:

In order to explore children's responses to the death of a sibling and their ability to report their reactions, the researcher will interview children aged 7 to 11. A non-experimental design will be used to gather data for this descriptive study.

The first sentence clearly indicates that this is a descriptive study and, by definition, non-experimental. What isn't clear is who these children are and what they'll be asked. Here's a more informative version:

To explore children's responses to the death of a sibling and determine their ability to report their reactions, a group of children aged 7–11 who have recently lost a brother or sister will be asked to describe their reactions to the death, in a structured interview.

Schematic Representation of the Design

It is often helpful to provide a schematic representation of the study design immediately following the overview. To draw the design after describing it may seem like telling the reader the same thing twice, just as naming the design does. But there is a difference. Labeling your design gives no additional information; in fact, you can name it without knowing what you're talking about or name one design while describing another. Besides, since different people use different labels for the same design, names may confuse readers even if you do know what you're talking about. But drawing the design gives additional information and thus clarifies and confirms for readers the impressions gained from the overview. The more complex the design the wiser it is to include the diagram.

Many research texts tell you how to draw and label your design. Here's an example. If you plan to assess compliance with medication-taking between an experimental group who are taught about medications and a comparison group who are not taught, you probably plan a pre- and posttest for the experimental group and two tests similarly separated in time for the comparison group. You would write:

The design may be represented as follows:

$O_1 \times O_2$
$O_1 \quad O_2$
$\times$ is the intervention
O_1 is the pretest (observation 1)
O_2 is the posttest (observation 2)

Some readers like to have both the independent and dependent variables labelled also. To do that write, "$\times$ is the independent variable, teaching about medications; O_1 is the pretest measuring the dependent variable, compliance in taking medications; and O_2 is the posttest measuring the dependent variable."

Hypotheses

Research texts usually describe the function and form of hypotheses in such a way that it seems easy to write them, at least from a distance. Close to one's own proposal, however, they often look tricky. The most important thing to remember about the wording of a hypothesis is that it always names some kind of expected measurable difference between two or more groups, or some kind of expected measurable association between two or more variables.

Hypotheses for Studies That Do Not Include an Intervention. Studies often predict relationships between variables when there is no intervention and a cause and effect relationship cannot be established. All of these studies use one of two types of hypotheses.

Type 1. *Non-Directional Hypotheses*
If you expect two variables to be associated but are not predicting the direction of the association, write the hypothesis this way:

Nurses' age will be associated with their attitudes toward pain control.

The formula is simple: "X will be associated with Y." It is the same no matter how many variables you include. Note that the hypothesis names the variables expected to be associated but does not indicate how they might be related. The variables are written as nouns, noun phrases, or noun clauses—nurses' age, nurses' attitudes toward pain control.

All variables must be clearly measurable. Age is measurable, of course, but either in the hypothesis itself or immediately following it you will have to indicate how attitude is to be determined. You might write:

> Nurses' age and level of education will be associated with the degree of comfort they feel in caring for terminally ill children, as determined by questionnaire.

Or, you could make a new sentence to follow the hypothesis:

> Degree of comfort will be determined by questionnaire.

Type 2. *Directional Hypotheses*

To predict the direction of the association between variables, you can write a hypothesis this way:

> Younger nurses will report more positive attitudes toward AIDS patients than older nurses.

You can say the same thing in several different ways:

> Older nurses will report more negative attitudes toward AIDS patients than younger nurses will.

> The younger the nurse, the more positive her reported attitude to AIDS patients will be.

> The older the nurse, the more negative her reported attitude to AIDS patients will be.

The formula is this:

> The more there is of X, the less there will be of Y,
> or
> The less there is of X, the more there will be of Y,

or
The more there is of X, the more there will be of Y,
     or
The less there is of X, the less there will be of Y.

You could construct the hypothesis in still another way:

Age will be negatively correlated with attitude toward AIDS patients.

The formula here is "X will be negatively (or positively) correlated with Y."

The first construction uses comparative phrases like "younger nurses" and "more positive attitude" to establish the direction of the association. The second construction uses nouns and indicates the direction by "negatively" or "positively."

Hypotheses for Studies That Include an Intervention. In a study with an intervention, the hypothesis predicts a difference between a group receiving the intervention and another group not receiving it; or between the change in scores, pre to post, of a group receiving the intervention and a group not receiving it; or between one group before and after the intervention; or between a group who receives one treatment and another group who receives a different treatment. You might write:

Patients who receive routine pain medications after surgery will report significantly less pain, as measured by questionnaire, than a matched control group receiving the same medications PRN.

The formula for the hypothesis is this:

Group A patients who receive X will have significantly more (or less) of Y than Group B patients who receive Z (or do not receive X).

The study may be simpler or more rigorous, but the form of the hypothesis remains the same. The variable expected to be affected by the treatment must be measurable and you must indicate how—either in the hypothesis (by saying, for example, "as measured by questionnaire") or in a separate sentence that follows the hypothesis.

Take this hypothesis, for example:

Patients who routinely receive at least two days of intensive care after surgery will develop significantly fewer complications than similar patients who are transferred to regular units from the recovery room.

Here the expected difference is in the number of complications. Number is clearly measurable but you will have to indicate to readers somewhere how you will define complications and what you will include under that heading.

If you compare the recipients of a treatment to themselves before and after, and also compare them to another group not receiving the treatment, the form is a little more complicated though the sense is basically the same. If the sentence gets too complicated split the hypothesis into two. Here's the combined form:

A group of patients with chronic back pain who use pain medication pumps to control pain will report significantly less pain with the pump than before using it, and significantly less pain than a comparison group receiving similar pain medications PRN.

Here are the separate forms:

Hypothesis 1—A group of patients with chronic back pain who use pain medication pumps to control pain will report significantly less pain with the pump than before using it.

Hypothesis 2—A group of patients with chronic back pain who use pain medication pumps to control pain will report significantly less pain than a comparison group receiving similar pain medications PRN.

If the difference being studied is a difference in change in scores between groups, pre and post, write the hypothesis this way:

The depression levels of a group of hospitalized mentally disturbed women who are taught assertiveness training will drop significantly more from pretest to posttest than the depression levels of a similar group not given assertiveness training.

If you expect the intervention to affect two or more dependent variables, it is wise to write a separate hypothesis for each expected difference, thus:

Hypothesis 1—A group of stroke patients who are assisted with regular exercise while still hospitalized will report significantly greater mobility six weeks after discharge than a group of similar patients who are not exercised while still hospitalized.

Hypothesis 2—A group of stroke patients who are assisted to exercise regularly while still hospitalized will show significantly lower depression levels six weeks after discharge than a group of similar patients who are not exercised while still hospitalized.

In a study with an intervention you may also predict some associations between outcomes of the intervention and variables you do not control, such as age, diagnosis, etc. For those hypotheses, use the form you'd use in studies without an intervention.

Formats for Hypotheses. Hypotheses do not need to be set off with a separate heading; they follow logically from the overview and design. Simply write a sentence to introduce them, like one of these:

The study hypotheses are as follows:
The study will test the following hypotheses:
It is hypothesized that . . .

With the first two introductions, the hypotheses themselves should be written as complete sentences. In the third, the hypotheses are clauses, separated by semicolons. It's a good idea to number your hypotheses if there are more than one or two.

In a proposal a hypothesis is usually stated in the future tense: "X *will be* associated with Y," "Group A *will have* better outcomes than Group B."

It is best not to state a hypothesis in the null form in your narrative. The null hypothesis has a statistical function, but it has no place in a narrative. Hypotheses represent your expectations, hopes, convictions. Always state them positively.

If you are predicting a difference between a group receiving an intervention and a comparison group, the experimental group should come first in the sentence: "Group A receiving X will have better outcomes than Group B not receiving X." And the difference between the groups should be expressed as a comparison: more than, less than, better than.

It is impossible to make the expected difference clear if you don't use a comparative form. Take this hypothesis, for example:

> A group of patients experiencing chronic pain will report a significant decrease in pain from pretest to posttest after practicing progressive relaxation when compared to a control group of patients not practicing relaxation.

This hypothesis does not make clear that the difference in pain between experimental and control group is expected to be greater after the intervention than before it. First, it sounds as though the experimental group will be compared only to itself from pretest to posttest; then suddenly there's the "when compared to a control group," which is very confusing. Compared to a control group when? How? With what expectation? The hypothesis should read:

> Patients experiencing chronic back pain who are taught progressive relaxation and practice regularly will report a significantly greater decrease in pain from pretest to posttest than will a control group of similar patients who do not practice relaxation.

Research Questions

If you are not making any predictions about what your study will show, you will probably have some specific questions you want to answer. If you have only one global question, it will be enough to make it clear in your purpose and probably repeat it in slightly different words in your overview. If your overall question is large and vague, however, then it must be broken down into more specific areas of interest. The research questions should come right after the overview. Introduce them in a sentence of this sort:

Specific questions for study are these:
Specifically, the study will attempt to answer these questions:
The research questions are as follows:

Then state the questions and number them if you like. For example, suppose you are interested in finding out whether nurses know enough about AIDS to care for and counsel AIDS patients adequately. Your research questions might be written this way:

1. How much do nurses know about the risk factors associated with AIDS?
2. How much do nurses know about the signs and symptoms of AIDS?
3. How much do nurses know about the prognosis and possible treatments for AIDS?
4. Is the nurse's age associated with overall knowledge of AIDS?

In writing research questions, the aim is to fall somewhere between too broad and too narrow. Be specific enough so that the answers to the questions won't be vague generalities, but don't be so nit-picking that you'll wind up with dozens of uncategorizable bits of information. And be sure that each question is clear and distinct from the others.

A good way to assess the adequacy and completeness of your research questions is to check them against the questionnaire or whatever instrument you'll be using to collect data. Do the research questions indicate clearly what variables the instruments will measure? Will those instruments provide answers to all the questions? Be sure the fit is good; if it is not, you may need to rewrite or add more questions.

Exploratory Questions.   In a study whose outcomes you are predicting, you will undoubtedly state hypotheses. But you may also have questions about additional variables and associations that you cannot predict. These exploratory questions come after the hypotheses. They should be introduced with a sentence like one of these:

The study will also explore the following:
The study will attempt to answer these additional questions:
The study will also provide exploratory data on the following:

Then the questions are stated just as in a study without hypotheses. Be sure there is no overlap between hypotheses and research questions; they must always be on different subjects. Research questions are *not* hypotheses written a different way. If you predict that "X will be related to Y," don't then ask, "Will X be related to Y?"

Definitions

Research texts explain that the concepts you use must be clear and that you must have an operational definition for each of your variables. If, for example, you are going to compare different methods of pain control, you must understand the various theoretical definitions of pain, the pain pathways and mechanisms, and the methods of action of pain medications and other treatments. You also have to have some way to measure pain in order to compare different methods of controlling it.

But gaining an understanding of the conceptual and operational definitions of variables and writing about these variables are not the same process. Writing is a public act in which you present readers with what *they* need to know in order to understand, not what *you* needed to do in order to clarify your own thinking.

When you write, the general rule is this: If you are using a term with a special or technical meaning — one that your audience cannot reasonably be expected to know — then define the term in context the first time you use it. It makes no sense to use a term for ten pages without defining it and then insert a section called "Definition of Terms" and define it there.

As a matter of fact, you are quite likely to define words informally when you first introduce them, without realizing that what you're doing is "definition." Take the term "pain." If you plan to study different methods of pain control, you will probably make it clear in the opening pages of your literature review how you're using the term. You do this by presenting various views of what pain is and how it operates, and indicating which of these views seems sound to you, i.e., what definition you plan to use.

Sometimes you need to be explicit about definition and if you do, don't wait; tell readers as soon as you define a term or mention another's definition that this is the meaning you've accepted. On occasion you'll need to give a more formal definition. Again, give it the first time you mention the word. If you don't need to tell readers what you mean by a concept or term the first time it appears, you don't ever need to tell them.

Many people feel they should have a section called "Definition of Terms," and sometimes they are hard pressed to find anything to put in it. So they define words that do not require definition (like "spouse") or they withhold information so that they can offer it later as definition. Never withhold information from readers when providing it can make reading easier. For example, if you plan to observe the adequacy of the instructions that registered nurses give patients about dealing with radiation side effects, don't talk generally about "nurses" or "nursing staff" throughout the literature review and in your purpose and overview statements and then in "Definitions" say, "A nurse is defined in this study as someone licensed and registered to practice nursing, an RN." Make it clear from the beginning that you plan to study RNs only, not LPNs or nurses' aides.

While the conceptual or theoretical definitions that people put in a section called "Definitions" should usually come in the literature review or in the overview of the study methods, the operational definitions should usually come with or immediately after the hypotheses.

An operational definition describes the procedure or process that allows you to use a term; in a proposal the function of the definition is to show how you will measure a variable. Suppose, for example, you are predicting that a group of dialysis patients who are taught stress management techniques will experience less anxiety than a group receiving no such instruction. Or you predict that anxiety will be lower among cancer patients who are informed in advance of the full range of side effects of radiation therapy than among patients who are uninformed. You plan to measure anxiety using a particular tool. That's your operational definition of anxiety and since it shows the reader how you'll be able to test the hypothesis, you need to give the information about the tool along with that hypothesis. To save it for a special section is to withhold a crucial piece of data from readers at the time they need it.

The other material seen in "Definitions" usually belongs among the criteria for sample selection. Take this "definition" for instance: "A critical care nurse is defined for the purpose of this study as a nurse employed on a critical care unit for at least six months, 16 to 40 hours per week." The term "critical care nurse" probably is clear to the audience; it should not need defining. And the length of time employed and hours worked are not part of a definition of critical care nurse; rather, they are among the criteria for the sample. For this study the investigator wants nurses who have worked on the unit long enough and worked enough shifts to have a good idea of what's been happening there — perfectly reasonable requirements, but they do not constitute a definition.

As these examples show, there's generally no reason to have a section called "Definition of Terms." If you are tempted to put together a set of definitions, ask yourself where the information belongs (in the introductory sections of your proposal, with the hypotheses, or in the section on sample criteria) and put it there.

Sometimes a thesis or dissertation committee will require a section called "Definition of Terms." That is because the committee views proposal writing as an exercise in thinking through and planning research, and part of that exercise is to show that you have conceptual and operational definitions for your variables. If you show the committee that you have in fact thought through the conceptualization and have adequate means of measuring your variables, you may be able to dispense with this section.

You can, for instance, produce a list of the terms you have defined and point to their definitions, whether in the literature review or with the hypotheses. You can argue then that thinking through research and writing a proposal are two different though overlapping activities, and it's better to use this proposal as an exercise in writing clearly about plans than as a demonstration of your thinking process. If your committee nonetheless requires a section on definitions, try putting it in an appendix. Then you make the information available without repeating in a special section of the narrative material you've provided elsewhere.

Setting

Description. The setting where you'll conduct your research should be described before you discuss the sample. First tell readers enough about that setting to make clear the extent to which your findings there will be generalizable to other settings. Indicate the type of setting: community hospital, health clinic, intensive care unit in a teaching and referral hospital, cancer center, psychiatric ward in a large university hospital, physician's office. Also mention the size, small, large, or, in the case of units or hospitals, give a bed capacity number; and note the location, in mid-South, West, Northwest, etc., indicating whether the setting is rural or urban.

If there are other aspects of the setting that may differ importantly from other settings, give those details too. For example, the type of provider and the socioeconomic level of the population served may affect the generalizability of the findings; therefore if you are going to conduct a study in a small rural southern health clinic serving mainly poor blacks and staffed by nurse practitioners with physician backup by phone, you need to be specific about those facts.

It is rarely necessary to name the particular setting. And if you do so in a proposal, you'll probably need to remove the information when you publish your findings, so it's as well to leave it out now. If you have limited contact with your thesis or dissertation committee members, however, it may be useful to name the agency in your proposal. If committee members have particular information about that setting they can give you helpful suggestions on how to proceed.

If you are using two different settings give parallel information on both, making clear the differences between them so readers can see how much of the territory you're covering. For example, you might write, "This study will be conducted in two health clinics. One, in the rural South, is staffed by two nurse practitioners with physician backup by phone; the other, in a northeastern city, is staffed by two physicians and six nurse practitioners."

If you have more than one setting, decide on a tag name for each and use it consistently. For example, the first time you refer to the clinic staffed only by nurse practitioners, you could call it "the nurse practitioner clinic (NP clinic)," and use "NP clinic" from then on. Tags should be short—their purpose is to save space and readers' time—and clear in their identification. Beware of meaningless labels such as "Setting A" and "Setting B," which tell nothing and require readers to remember which is which or constantly look back to see.

Make sure your tags fit grammatically into the narrative. Never say "the staffed only by NPs clinic." It's worth spending a little time trying to think of good labels for settings (or different groups). Good tags, like good titles, may only help you a little, but bad ones can hurt you a lot.

Standard Procedures. After you've described the setting briefly, review any standard procedures for patients or clients or others you'll be sampling in this setting, if those procedures are relevant to your study. For example, if you're going to look at the adequacy of the information on side effects that nurses give chemotherapy patients in an outpatient cancer clinic, or if you will intervene to provide additional information to patients in the clinic, you need to review the standard procedure for patients as they go through the clinic: "Patients check in, have blood counts made, see a nurse who weighs them and checks their temperature, see the physician, get intravenous drugs from the chemotherapy nurse, get a new appointment, then leave."

If that information is not relevant to your study, omit it. For instance, if you are going to survey patients about the side effects they experience after treatment, it probably doesn't matter how they go through the clinic. Remember that the standard procedures of the setting are not part of your study; that's why they belong with the setting description, not with the description of your research procedures.

Numbers of Subjects Ordinarily Seen. It is important to explain why you think you will get the numbers you need for your sample in this setting. If you expect to collect data on the prenatal clients the NP handles alone in a clinic over a period of two months, you will doubtless have checked with the clinic to find out how many pregnant women usually come to the clinic over a two-month period. Pass that information on to readers, so they can conclude with you that the setting will supply what is needed.

Exceptions. Many mailed surveys do not require a description of a setting for the obvious reason that the respondents are in all sorts of settings. In that case, omit the section titled "Setting" and simply list the sources of the sample in your section on the sample.

Proposals for field studies may need to include more extensive descriptions of the setting than other studies, because it is not clear ahead of time which aspects are going to be important. Content analyses have no setting, strictly speaking. In cases like these, you have to decide what information readers need. If they need more, give it; if less, omit it.

Sample

Criteria and Method of Selection.   To evaluate your research plan, proposal readers need to know what population you are sampling, what your criteria are for including subjects (or events, observations, records) in the sample, and how you'll select those subjects (whether randomly, purposely, by accident or convenience). You can provide this information in several ways. Begin your description, however, by explaining what the sampling unit will be, if that will not be clear from other statements.

Here is a simple way to describe the sample criteria and the method of selection:

> The criteria for inclusion in the study are as follows:
> 1. Diagnosis of hypertension
> 2. Age over 18
> 3. Ability to read at an eighth grade level
> 4. Consent to participate

Coming after your description of the setting, this list makes it clear that you will not select a sample randomly but will take all those in the setting who meet the three basic criteria of the study and consent to participate. In a list like this, every item must have the same grammatical structure, usually nouns and noun phrases.

If the pieces of information won't fit together easily in a list, try using a sentence. For example, you can say:

> Clinic clients over 18 who have a diagnosis of hypertension and are overweight will be included in the study if they can read at an eighth grade level and consent to participate.

Like the list, this sentence indicates that you will make no effort at random selection but will take everyone who meets your criteria. Unlike the list, the sentence form allows you to use different grammatical constructions and also to distinguish between the basic characteristics of the population you're sampling (that is, the diagnosis, age limits, weight status) and those criteria for inclusion that are practical and ethical (ability to read and consent to participate).

If your criteria are more complex, you can set them up in a series of sentences, the first giving the basic criteria, the second listing specific exclusions, and the last dealing with practical and ethical concerns. For example,

> The subjects will be overweight clinic patients aged 18–65 with a diagnosis of hypertension. Those who are taking medications to control the hypertension or who have complicating problems such as diabetes will be excluded from the study. Only those subjects who can read at an eighth grade level and who consent to participate will be included in the sample.

Again, it is clear that you will make no random selection among those eligible but take all who consent and can read.

If you plan to use any form of probability sampling, you must make the method clear. If the population you are sampling is easily described you can give both the criteria for inclusion and the method of sampling in one sentence. For example:

> Using a table of random numbers, a sample of 500 registered nurses will be selected from lists of registered nurses currently licensed to practice in the states of North Carolina, Kansas, and Oregon.

That sentence makes clear what your criterion for inclusion is, what places you'll draw from, and how you'll get a random sample. It's also going to be obvious from your earlier overview and this description that you'll be mailing a survey to your sample and that completion and return of the questionnaire will constitute consent.

Sometimes one sentence is not enough. In such cases give the criteria first, in a list or in a sentence; then describe the method you'll use to select the sample and obtain consent to participate, if consent is required. Finally, explain why you are using a particular method, unless that will be immediately clear to readers. Suppose, for example, you plan to survey every third person with Type II diabetes who comes to your clinic over a period of one year. You mght describe the sample like this:

> A systematic sample will be drawn from patients aged 18–65 with Type II diabetes who come to the clinic over a period of one year. Those who are more than 20% overweight or have significant hypertension will be excluded. Every third patient meeting the criteria will be asked to participate. Using every third patient, a sample of approximately 100 is expected in this time period, which is sufficient for the analyses planned.

Naming the type of sample is a bit like naming the type of design. It's no substitute for describing how you'll select the sample. But if it seems helpful to include the name, do so.

Numbers.   The description of the sample should include the number of people you are expecting and the reasoning behind this expectation: either the setting will supply them in the ordinary course of events or you'll collect data until you get them. Your description of the setting may have prepared readers by giving the number of people in the category you're interested in who are seen in this setting over a typical time period. In that case, just conclude here by saying, "A sample of 59 (or 590, or whatever) is expected during the data collection period of six months (or whatever the period is)."

If you have not prepared readers, you can give the number you expect in the opening sentence of your sample description and explain later:

> A random sample of 200 will be drawn from among those nurses who meet the following criteria:

Or you can conclude your sample description by saying how many people you intend to include and why you expect them. Or simply say, "Data will be collected until 50 people have been entered into the study."

Groups.   If you plan to include two or more groups in your study, tell how you will assign people to these groups; do this after you describe your sample criteria but before you explain how many subjects you expect. Suppose, for example, you plan to assign your sample members randomly to either a group of patients who receive relaxation training or a group who do not. First give the criteria for inclusion in the study; then describe the method you'll use to assign sample members to either the experimental or control group; and finally, tell how many you expect in each group and why, or indicate that you will collect data until some target number is reached.

Perhaps you plan to collect data on satisfaction with nursing care from patients on three units who receive routine nursing care; then you will institute a system of primary nursing on these units and collect similar data on patients who receive the new type of care. First you'll give the criteria for inclusion in the study and any specific exclusions. Then you might say:

> Those patients admitted to the units in June and July who meet the study criteria and consent to participate will constitute the comparison group. Those patients meeting the criteria who are admitted in August and September, after the institution of primary nursing, and who consent to participate will constitute the experimental group.

Next say how many you expect in each group; if you haven't already made it clear why, make that clear now.

The description of your groups prepares readers for what's coming: the intervention. If there is to be no intervention and there are no groups, go straight from the description of the sample and the number of subjects you expect to the data you'll collect on them.

Consent to Participate.   Any nursing research done on human beings requires their consent, and you should mention this consent as one of the criteria for inclusion in the study. The information on how you gain subjects' consent is given later, in the section headed "Procedure." As mentioned earlier, you do not need to mention consent as a criterion for the sample when you are conducting a survey in which subjects have the option of returning a questionnaire or not. In such cases, completion and return constitute consent to participate in the study. You point that out to readers in your section on "Procedure."

Sample or Procedure?   People often confuse the description of the sample with the description of their research procedures, and then some pieces of information appear twice. Look at this description of a sample, for instance:

> The sample will include all of the children at the day camp aged 7 to 11 who have parental permission to participate in the study. A letter explaining the study and consent information will be given to each child in that age range to take home and return if the parents grant permission for the child to participate.

The first sentence gives the criteria for inclusion in the study: age 7–11 and parental permission. But the second sentence describes the procedure for approaching individuals and gaining their consent to participate; that information does not belong in the description of the sample.

To avoid confusion and overlap, remember that in the section on the sample you give criteria and method of selection for the sample as a whole, while in "Procedure" you tell how you will approach each individual, find out whether that individual meets the criteria, and ask for agreement to participate.

Intervention

The intervention—the experiment or treatment you'll give or the change you'll make and evaluate—should be explained step by step, in chronological order, or piece by piece, if the treatment or program is in sections. For example, suppose you plan to teach cardiac patients stress reduction through progressive muscle relaxation. First tell what you will teach them and how, then say what you will do to reinforce the teaching and see whether they've learned. Or suppose you plan to institute a system of primary nursing on three units in the hospital. Say what the new system will be like: first, what the primary nurse will do that is observably different from routine care, and then what the other nurses working with the primary nurse will do that is different from ordinary team nursing. In short, explain each part of the new system.

Theoretically, the intervention should be described in enough detail so that someone else can put it into effect if you are unable to carry out your proposed research. But the detailed information doesn't have to go into the "Methods" section; you can put it in the appendix. Say you have developed a series of lesson plans for the school nurse to use in teaching elementary school children about smoking, nutrition, alcohol, and drugs. You do not need to give the complete plans in the body of the proposal; just describe generally the content of the four parts and indicate how that content will be presented. Save the details for an appendix. But do give enough information in the narrative to make the intervention understandable.

The more complex and precise the intervention, the more details are necessary in the narrative. A good way to find out whether your description is complete enough is to read it aloud to a couple of colleagues and ask them if they can imagine how to carry the program through. If they are puzzled you need to add more details.

Always describe the intervention before you describe what you will do to a comparison group. For example, if you are comparing some new type of nursing care with routine care, describe the new care first; then describe the routine care that a comparison group will receive.

After describing the intervention and telling what, if anything, a comparison group will receive, add a sentence giving the sequence of data collection to prepare readers for your description of data collection tools, which should come next. If you have a pretest/posttest design, for example, you might say that the two groups will be pretested, then the experimental group will receive the treatment while the comparison group receives no treatment (or routine treatment), and finally both groups will be posttested. If you'll collect data on the comparison group first, then institute the experimental care, say so. If you plan to give the treatment to the comparison group after you've collected data, mention that fact last.

Occasionally an intervention is based on or modified by assessment data collected from a group who then serve as a comparison group. If you plan to base your intervention on such data, the description of the intervention and sequence of data collection will be a little different. Let's say you plan to collect data from patients on what they find stressful in the ICU, then teach the nursing staff about these stressors in an effort to assist them to reduce stress, then ask a second group of patients what they find stressful in the unit. Begin with a general description of the data you'll collect from the first group, but don't go into detail; save the detail for data collection tools. Next say how you'll use the data to design your intervention and describe the intervention as fully as you can at this stage; then tell what data you'll collect on the group who receive the intervention.

Whatever the order of your points, watch out for confusion with procedure. To avoid putting the same information in two places, think of the intervention as a standard program you need to describe, not your own plan of action. In other words, describe the intervention as a set of operations that will exist whether you actually carry them out or not. Then later in your "Procedure" section, tell readers how you plan to put these standard operations into practice.

Variables and Their Measurement

Introduction.   Begin the section about your data collection tools by telling readers what you will collect data on. Name the variables on which the study will focus and say what other information you'll seek. Then list the instruments you'll use to collect the data, and, finally, say when you plan to collect data if you will do so at more than one point. Suppose, for example, you plan to hold eight weeks of group therapy sessions for a group of elderly depressed men and women and you will compare their depression levels before and after therapy with the depression levels of a group who receive anti-depressants but no therapy. You're also going to collect data on other factors that might be associated with depression such as recent losses and current social supports, age, socioeconomic status, and infirmities. You need to tell readers in the introductory paragraph that you will measure the depression levels of the treatment and comparison groups using a particular scale or scales, before and after the therapy period, and will also collect data on age, infirmities, and other factors possibly associated with depression.

If you will use two or more measurement tools, name them all in the introductory paragraph; then when you describe them, do so in the same order you introduced them. It's wise to begin with the more objective and precise and move toward more subjective and imprecise measures. Thus, physiological measures requiring technical equipment should be described first; then scheduled observations, and finally questionnaires or interview schedules. If you are using two or more measures of one type (two scales or questionnaires) introduce and describe them in the order of their importance, not in the order you'll administer them. This tells your proposal readers immediately what you consider most important; further, it will save time when you move from proposal to report, for then you will want to prepare for and present your most important findings first.

Physiological Measures.   When you measure a physiological parameter, first say what you'll measure, then tell what instrument you'll use, how it functions, and precisely how you will use it if there are any possible variations. For example, will you measure blood pressure or lung capacity after exercise or at rest? What position will patients be in when you take their temperature? Next say at what times you'll take the measurement and how you'll record the data. If you plan more than one physiological measurement, describe the process you'll use for each measure in a separate paragraph, moving from most important to least important.

Scheduled Observations.   If you plan scheduled observations, first say as precisely as possible what you'll observe, whether it's eating habits or sleeping patterns in the ICU, urinary output, or nonverbal communication. If the phenomenon you'll observe is clearly delineated and can be measured precisely, like urinary output, you need only say how you'll collect and record the data.

But suppose you're observing facial expressions. Which ones will you look for, and how do you define them? You might decide to count the number of times a woman in labor grimaces or closes her eyes or gives other facial indicators of pain. Say precisely what it is you're looking at, or how you'll interpret what you see if it's not precisely defined. That is, you must tell how you'll define and categorize the units of observation. Then describe how you'll collect the data: Will you watch this patient continuously for five minutes, will you film an interview, will you have every nurse who enters the room observe and record on a checklist the variables you're interested in? Tell readers what you'll do and how you'll record what you find.

If you are not going to make the observations yourself, tell how you will instruct the people who observe for you. And if there are two or more observers, say what you'll do to ensure that they interpret and record what they see in the same way or as nearly the same as possible.

Questionnaires and Interviews.   Although writers usually supply sufficient detail about planned physiological measurements and observations, they are sometimes tempted to omit the details about a questionnaire or scale because the whole thing can be included in the appendix. But appendixes are for reference, not to make up for laziness. (See Part Four, pages 191–192, for a discussion of the contents of appendixes.) Always give the flavor of a questionnaire in the body of the proposal; don't make readers turn elsewhere to get even a taste of what you'll do.

If you plan to question people about vignettes, describe the stories first, then discuss the questions you'll ask. If yours is a straight questionnaire, first name its subject area, tell the number of questions it contains or otherwise indicate its length, and list the subtopics. For instance, a questionnaire asking families their concerns about keeping a dying patient at home might include several questions on the need for various types of equipment, some questions on the need for resource personnel, and questions about psychological support and relief. Each is a major subtopic of the questionnaire. By describing them, you give readers a sense of what your data will cover and how the data will be categorized. You also prepare for the description of scoring if you have a scale composed of several subscales.

It is helpful to include sample questions (if it's a formal questionnaire, you'll include the whole thing in the appendix) so readers can see just what a respondent is facing. But don't stick the questions in like raisins in a bun; paraphrase them to fit smoothly into your narrative.

After you've given readers a taste of the questionnaire, indi-

cate how the respondent will answer the questions: Does the respondent mark on a scale, answer yes or no, choose among several
options, or are the questions open-ended? If you have more than
one type of question, describe each type separately and say how
many questions of each type you will ask. Then explain how the
answers will be scored or totaled, or what weight will be attached
to them, and how they will be compared or combined. If this is a
scale, give full information on the scoring method unless it is so
intricate that it will overwhelm readers. (In that case, explain the
details in an appendix.) Also give the possible range of scores for
the scale and mention any norms.

If you plan interviews, describe the interview schedule just as
you would describe a questionnaire. Tell the kinds of questions
you will ask, give some examples, say how the questions are to be
answered and how you'll categorize and record the data. If you are
not doing the interviews, tell how the interviewers will be trained.
And if two or more people will conduct the interviews, explain how
you'll establish interrater reliability for their categorization of
the data.

In describing a questionnaire or interview schedule you developed yourself, use the present tense to discuss numbers and types
of questions and use the future tense to say what respondents will
do with the questions and what you will do with their responses.
For example, if you have developed a questionnaire to find out
what patients scheduled for a CT scan for the first time know about
the procedure and what they feel about it in anticipation, you
might write:

> The questionnaire begins with an open-ended question asking the
> respondents what they know about the CT scan and the source of the
> information. Then follow eight multiple-choice questions exploring
> the respondents' knowledge of the purpose of the CT scan, required
> preparation for the scan, the procedure itself, and the way a patient is
> likely to feel during the procedure. A final open-ended question asks
> respondents what they feel anticipating the procedure. Responses to
> the open-ended knowledge question will be categorized as reflecting
> no information or misinformation, some information, and good in-
> formation. Responses to the multiple-choice questions will be simi-
> larly categorized. The anxiety expressed by the respondent in the
> final question will be categorized as absent or minor, moderate or
> extreme. Level of information will then be examined in relation to
> level of anxiety.

If you are using a questionnaire or scale developed and tested by someone else, treat it as a standard procedure and discuss it entirely in the present tense. For example, you might write:

> Respondents are presented statements, and they indicate the degree of their agreement or disagreement with each on a Likert-type scale. A total score is derived to indicate each respondent's overall satisfaction (or overall depression, or overall anxiety, etc.).

When you have described the questionnaire fully, add a sentence telling how it will be administered: mailed, read aloud, handed out and completed on the spot, or collected at a later date. Next indicate how long it will take a respondent to complete it.

Then and only then should you report on the tool's validity and reliability—validity before reliability. Speak first of content validity, then give the data on concurrent validity, and finally construct validity. When you come to reliability, first give the information on internal consistency, then on test-retest reliability, and finally, if relevant, the data on interrater reliability.

For other people's instruments, you often have all the information you need on validity and reliability. If you have some but not all of it, first describe what you have, then indicate what is missing. If the data are not relevant to your use of the tool, don't mention them.

If this is your own instrument, mention any experts you have consulted or will consult to establish its validity, indicating the type of expertise, not the names; don't forget to mention the literature if you have used that as a basis for developing the tool. Then describe any pilot test you have conducted or will conduct to ensure that the questionnaire is clearly written, measures what it is intended to measure, and can be completed in a reasonable time.

When you've described how you'll collect data on all your independent and dependent variables, conclude by indicating what data you'll collect on those characteristics of the sample that might affect your other findings—age, race, socioeconomic status, type of educational preparation, diagnosis, or whatever else might be relevant. Put this type of data last even if you plan to obtain it first, for unless this is a survey focusing on demographic data, these are the least important data you'll collect.

When you finish this section on data collection, check the

description of your measurements against the hypotheses or research questions you listed earlier, to be sure that you've shown how you'll get the data needed to answer the questions or test the hypotheses.

Anecdotal Data. When you collect quantifiable data through physiological measurements, scheduled observations, or interviews, you record the information as a matter of course. Qualitative data, if planned for, are also routinely recorded. But anecdotal data, because they are unplanned for, often go unrecorded. And alas, what makes that kind of information useful is the very thing that the memory cannot hold for long: concrete particulars. If you don't write down the unexpected or the confirming detail when you observe it or when the subject tells you about it, you'll forget. So plan to record every observation and anecdote that strikes you in the course of your study, even if you don't mention it in your proposal. It takes a little time to do, but you'll have a wealth of human information later to flavor your numbers, spice up your discussion, or help you understand unexpected findings. This kind of data will not only enrich your report but may also provide the basis for further studies or case histories.

Procedure

Access to the Sample. The section titled "Procedure" shows readers your plan of action. It should be organized exactly as you'll carry out the plans, step by step, in chronological order. First describe how you'll get access to the settings you've selected and to subjects in those settings, how you'll identify subjects, and how you'll approach them. You may need to indicate what permissions you already have and what permissions are still to be gained. Also tell readers about any institutional review boards for protection of human subjects to which you have sent or will send a proposal.

Protection of Rights of Human Subjects. To protect the rights of human subjects, you need to explain your study to potential subjects and assure them that participation is voluntary and they have a right to refuse to participate or to withdraw at any time. Further, they need to be told that withdrawal will not affect their care if they are patients, their grades if they are students, or their performance evaluations if they are employees. In addition, you need to assure them confidentiality and anonymity and tell them how you will protect their privacy. If your study procedures will bring any risk to participants, you must point out those risks, as well as the potential benefits of participation.

To make clear to readers that you will take adequate measures to protect human subjects' rights, you must indicate in your proposal whether or not the study procedures will bring risks to subjects and, if they do, why those risks are justified. Usually that means describing both the risks and the benefits of the study. Next, you must tell readers the information that you will provide to potential subjects and the assurances you will give to participants. If you do not plan to tell participants the true nature of the study, make that clear to readers and explain why. If you plan to offer any incentives or use any compulsions to gain participation, they too must be explained. If you do not need subjects' consent because you will only be studying charts or documents, make that clear as well.

Next describe the method you will use to ensure confidentiality and anonymity and then tell how subjects will give their consent, whether by signing a consent form, completing and returning the questionnaire, or whatever. In an appendix provide a copy of the information you will give potential subjects, and a copy of the consent form (see Part Four, pages 191–192, on appendixes).

The Research Process.   If you plan an intervention and will give a pretest, indicate when, where, and how the pretest will be given; then say when, where, and how the intervention will be carried out, and by whom. Suppose, for example, you will pretest and then teach a group of hospitalized hypertensive patients about diet and medications before their discharge. Will they be pretested and then taught immediately, or taught some time later? Will the teaching be a part of routine discharge instructions? Or will it be separate and occur sooner? Will you teach the patients? If not, who will? Will the teaching be done in the patient's room? With family members present? If not in the room, where? Give readers all the details you can about the schedule and arrangements, but don't describe the content of the teaching program; you've already presented the intervention.

Next give the details about posttests. Suppose you'll test these same patients' knowledge of medications on their first follow-up clinic visit. How will you get in touch with them? Where will you give the posttest? How will you fit it into the patient's appointment schedule?

If you have an experimental and a comparison group, always give the procedure for the experimental group first, then tell in which parts of the study the comparison group will participate. If they will receive the treatment after data collection is complete, say so.

If you plan no intervention, say when, where, and how you will collect data. Don't repeat the information about data collection tools that you've already given readers; just say how those tools will be administered to each individual subject. For example, after you've gained consent from a subject, you might first take his or her blood pressure, then ask him or her to fill out a questionnaire on recent life changes then and there, while you sit by ready to clarify or answer questions. Perhaps then you will remain available to discuss any concerns. Or perhaps you will hand the subject a questionnaire and ask him or her to mail it back to you when it is complete. This is the kind of information you need to give in "Procedure."

For interviews, it's sometimes difficult to decide where the standard interview schedule ends and the procedure for carrying it out begins, so you may have a bit of overlap. Don't worry about it; too much is better than too little information.

The "Methods" section should conclude with plans for follow-up or extension of the study if you do not get the sample you need in the allotted time for data collection. Do not talk in this section about how you will analyze your data. That information comes in the next section.

Chapter 5

Plans for Analysis and Use

This section of the proposal is by necessity the sketchiest, since the way you analyze your data depends in part on what you get, and the uses of the findings depend on what they are. If you knew already what they'd be, you'd have no reason for doing the study. Even so, you can say some things about analysis and use, for you know approximately what you can and cannot do with the types of data you'll collect, and you know how you hope your study will help solve the original problem or answer the initial question.

Begin by describing your plans for analysis based on the research questions or hypotheses. First say what you'll do to describe the data, starting with the sample and then moving to the results of physiological measures, observations, and on to questionnaire or interview data or scores. Indicate whether you will present frequency distributions and what tables you anticipate. If you draw up dummy tables for this section, you'll make some of your later work easier while giving proposal readers a clearer idea of what the outcomes might look like. (Suggestions for constructing tables are in Part Two, pages 103–104. More thorough information can be found in the APA style manual.)

Next tell how you'll analyze the data to answer your research questions or test your hypotheses. What kinds of statistical techniques will be appropriate? What will you need to do to the data to apply these techniques? It's helpful to discuss the analysis for each hypothesis or research question separately. Then talk about any possible further analyses you foresee.

After describing your plans for analysis, discuss the uses you expect the findings to have for theory development, further research, and practice, in that order. Present only the uses you can see clearly or imagine. You may have given some of your ideas about uses at the conclusion of the literature review; an overlap is all right, but the discussion here should be more substantial.

Always discuss the uses for practice last and do so in connection with a discussion of the limitations of your study. Say what will get in the way of implementing your findings in the real world—what will limit the generalizability of the findings from one setting to another, from your sample to the population, from this population to others. Point out what you can do in the analysis to deal with the limitations of your design or sampling method, but acknowledge any shortcomings that your analysis cannot overcome. Then conclude in a positive way by saying how useful the outcomes will be in spite of their limitations.

PART TWO

Writing a Thesis, Dissertation, or Research Report

Chapter 6

General Outline

Betty L. McMullen
University Lake Apts.
200 Barnes Street
Carrboro, N. C. 27510

There are those who think the thesis, the dissertation, the complete research report are a waste of energy and should be eliminated. These lengthy exercises are almost never publishable, the argument goes, and science would be better served if researchers omitted them and instead wrote articles that would make their findings available more quickly and to more people.

You may well agree that writing a lengthy report of your research will be a tremendous energy drain, but if you wrote a proposal and had your study approved, you are likely now to owe someone an accounting: a thesis or dissertation committee, an agency that funded your study, or an organization that gave you access to subjects.

Fortunately, a report is not as hard to write as a proposal because the literature review and the methods section in the proposal can usually be inserted in the report with only minor changes. New thinking and writing are necessary mainly in the sections that present and discuss your findings.

Here's the general outline for a research report, thesis, or dissertation. Those three may differ in complexity, but their format and organization are essentially the same, so for the sake of simplicity, the generic term "report" will be used.

Report Outline

I. Rationale for the study (introduction and review of the literature)

   A. The problem, question, or theory tested

   B. Work already done on the problem or question, or prior tests of the theory

   C. Shortcomings or gaps in the work already done

   D. The purpose of the study being reported

II. Methods

   A. The design of the present study (overview, hypotheses, and research questions)

   B. Setting and sample

   C. Intervention, if applicable

   D. Variables and their measurement (data collection tools)

   E. Research procedure

III. Findings

   A. Description of the sample

   B. Description of the study findings

   C. Hypothesis testing, if applicable

   D. Additional or exploratory analyses

IV. Discussion and conclusions

   A. Summary of major findings

   B. The general meaning of the findings and their relation to previous work

   C. Limitations on the generalizability of the findings

   D. Ways further research can overcome these limitations

   E. Usefulness of the findings for theory development

   F. Implications for practice

When the basic outline of the research report doesn't suit your purposes, alter it. For example, the outline of "Methods" given above may seem illogical if you gathered data on a group of subjects, designed an intervention on the basis of the data, and then collected more data on another group of subjects who experienced the intervention. With a design like that, a more logical organization of "Methods" is this:

II. Methods
   A. Design of the study
   B. Setting and samples
   C. Data collection tools for the first set of subjects
   D. Procedures for first set of subjects
   E. Findings from first data collection
   F. Intervention
   G. Data collection tools and procedures for second set of subjects (only the differences from tools and procedures for first set)

There are other cases when the complexity of your design or the complications of the world make the standard organization untenable. In such cases follow the logic of the study and modify the standard outline to suit it.

The easiest way to compose a research report is to begin with your findings. After you write that section, revise the section on methods, and, next, the review of the literature. Save the discussion section for last. Here, however, we'll take up each of the four sections in order, in separate chapters: you can skip around and read the chapters in the order you need them.

Although a research report is usually preceded by an abstract, the abstract cannot be written until the report is complete. Some suggestions for writing an abstract are included in Part Four (pages 192–196).

Chapter 7

Rationale (Introduction and Literature Review)

The literature review for a report is usually almost identical to that in the proposal. In part, that's because of practical constraints. By the time you get to the report, you're hurrying to meet a graduate school's or funding agency's deadline, you still have to write up the findings and figure out what they mean, so there's little or no time to redo the introductory material.

Usually there's no great need to do so, anyway, since the background for the study remains much the same. Besides, unless the report will be published as a monograph, which is unlikely, you will be rewriting material that will for the most part have to be thrown out when you move to an article. However, some changes in this section are usually required to make the parts of your report hang together, and there may be new studies you need to include. So it's not enough to skim the review; you need to reread, rethink your logic, and make whatever revisions are necessary to update the review and deal with any problems.

Introduction

In a research proposal the literature review sometimes begins with a four- or five-paragraph introduction that is like an abstract (see pages 192–196) of the review. If your proposal contained these introductory paragraphs, you must now decide whether you still need them, given that your report will be preceded by an abstract of the full study.

If the literature reviewed is very complex and you have pulled together a lot of material that might at first seem tangential to your aims, you may still wish to include a few opening paragraphs that introduce readers to the problem or question you studied, briefly mention the work done on the problem to date, and conclude with an overview of your study or its purpose. If the introduction to the proposal included any other material, omit it. Statements about the usefulness or significance of the research, for example, come at the end of a research report, not in the opening paragraphs; and the introduction should not contain hypotheses or research questions. Obviously, if you needed no introduction to the literature review in your proposal, you don't need one in the report.

Revising the Literature Review

New Studies. Before you begin revising the literature review, go back to the library to make sure nothing more has been published since you began your study. If there is something new, you must include it. While one or two new studies may have appeared, in most cases they will not be directly relevant to your research and you can easily insert a sentence or two about them in the middle of the literature review before your discussion of directly related work. Two types of studies can cause problems, however: (1) studies similar to yours that have produced *different* findings, and (2) studies similar to yours that have produced *similar* findings.

If a new study was similar but produced different findings, you can discuss it with other closely related work (as if you'd known of it all along), pointing out its shortcomings or lack of generalizability and the consequent need for further study. Or you can introduce it in the last paragraph of your literature review, noting that it is a new study, like this:

> The present study examined associations between continuation of treatment and social supports among a group of male and female

hypertensives, over a five-year period. A study by Rutledge and Hudson (1985), reported after this study began, found no association between social supports and compliance or continuation in treatment, but that study used only cross-sectional data. This longitudinal study examined supports and continuation in treatment at ten points over the five-year period.

Whenever you discuss the new study, do so in such a way that it adds to the rationale for your own study (as the example above does), or at the very least does not detract from your rationale.

If a new study produced findings similar to those you're reporting, you can discuss it with other closely related work near the end of the literature review. But you must point out the study's shortcomings to explain why yet another study was needed, or point to the differences between that study and your own. Or you can treat the new study as confirming your directions. In that case write about it in the paragraph that presents the purpose of your own study, like this:

> This study was designed to compare anxiety and depression after surgery between two groups of patients: one treated before surgery with a drug to reduce recall of surgery, and the other group taught relaxation techniques before surgery. A study by Jones and Smith (1985), reported after this study began, found that anxiety levels of patients taught relaxation were higher than those treated pharmacologically, adding support to the hypotheses of the present study. These hypotheses were as follows.

In the worst of all possible worlds some new study has appeared whose author expected to find what you expected to find. That author didn't find it and you didn't, either. The author explains why, and now you've discovered the same explanation on your own. For example, suppose you were expecting that a teaching program on ways to cope with pain would bring about a change in pain control behaviors among your sample of patients with chronic back pain. You did the teaching but you found no change. Now a new study has appeared reporting more or less the same intervention with the same type of patient population. That author also found no change, and in the discussion points out that it was unrealistic to expect people with long-ingrained habits to change them after a short teaching program; the author notes further that the depression and hopelessness that often accompany chronic pain must somehow be dealt with before people can be expected to change. You've come to the same conclusions. It is probably best to introduce this new study in the discussion of your findings. Point out that it is new, compare findings, and discuss the explanations the two of you have produced, then conclude that this other study reinforces what you have discovered.

The Thrust of the Review.   When you write a research proposal, you have certain expectations about what you'll find, and these are consciously or unconsciously reflected in your review of the literature. Thus, the review points readers in the direction of your hopes. If you then find what you hoped to find, the literature review will continue to point readers in the right direction. But if you don't find what you are looking for, the literature review will have the wrong thrust for your report.

Suppose, for example, you expected to find that a group of anxious, elderly women in a nursing home would become significantly less anxious after eight weeks of group therapy. In the proposal your literature review established the basis for your hypothesis by pointing to studies that would lead one to expect a reduction in anxiety as an outcome of group therapy. But when you did the research you found no significant difference in anxiety before and after therapy. At the same time, you found that confusion, which you also assessed along the way, seemed to be considerably less after the therapy. You now speculate that the attention given in therapy, along with the need to focus on group interactions, had something to do with this.

In other words, your findings and conclusions are quite useful, but they are not what you expected them to be. The original literature review in your proposal will not lead readers to these findings; rather, it points in one direction while your findings and discussion go in another. That will give the report a disjointed appearance, so you may need to refocus the final pages of the literature review. For example, instead of discussing closely related studies in a way that would lead readers to expect group therapy to reduce anxiety measurably, you might indicate merely that other studies of this question were not conclusive and another trial was needed. You might also add a paragraph pointing out that confusion often accompanies anxiety in the elderly, and note that no studies have examined the effect of therapy on confusion in this population. The first change neutralizes the original literature review so that it does not raise the wrong expectations. The second change lays the groundwork for your findings about confusion.

The more open the original literature review is to the unexpected and the less definitely it points in a particular direction, the less you will have to revise it if your study turns in a different direction from the one in which you began.

Time and Tenses. The concluding sentences of the literature review in your proposal probably stressed the need for further research. Now you need to rewrite those sentences to reflect that the further research has been done. For example, suppose you tested the effectiveness of deliberative nursing in helping a large sample of cancer patients control their pain. To introduce your purpose you concluded the description of the studies done before yours with statements like these:

> While the studies reported here had encouraging results, their small samples make generalization inadvisable. To test the effectiveness of deliberative nursing actions in controlling pain among cancer patients, further research is needed with larger samples randomly assigned to treatment and control groups.

That's the study you just did. Obviously, you don't want to begin a report describing that study by saying "further research is needed." Rewrite the sentences to more appropriately introduce your work, like this, for example:

> This study was designed to extend the research on the use of deliberative nursing to help patients control pain. Using a large sample of cancer patients with bony metastases, randomly assigned to treatment and control groups, the study explored the effectiveness of a specific set of deliberative nursing actions on patients' ability to pinpoint what was needed to control their pain.

Thus, you give the purpose of your study and indicate how it was designed to overcome the limitations of the earlier studies. Everything is now said in the past tense, because the study you are reporting is not beginning, it's complete.

Most of the statements about what you were setting out to do or what you expected were written in the future tense in the proposal. Now, they must be put into the past tense. If you're alert to these problems, they are generally easy to solve. In rewriting your literature review, the major enemy is carelessness — overlooking the sentence that's still in the future tense, for instance, or the paragraph that leads readers in the wrong direction. Close reading is your best weapon against that enemy.

Intended Uses.   In a research proposal the literature review often concludes with several paragraphs or even several pages on the significance or potential usefulness of the data being sought. That material should be omitted in the literature review for the report. Save all talk about the importance of the findings until you present them.

Chapter 8

Methods Section for
Research Reports

In a research report the section describing your methods is very similar to the one in the proposal, and it is organized exactly the same. The overview is first, followed by hypotheses or research questions or both; then comes the description of setting and sample, the intervention if applicable, and next the description of data collection tools; the research procedure is last. (See Part One, pages 36–42, for outlines of the methods section for various research designs.)

A research *proposal*, however, describes the methods you intend to use; a research *report* describes the methods you actually used, and the two are not necessarily the same. Sometimes, though, what you proposed to do and what you did turn out to be very similar and it's easy then to write the section on methods for the report. You can simply lift this section from the proposal, put it into the past tense, and edit it slightly to reflect the minor changes that almost inevitably occur. But sometimes things don't work out as planned. You find in your pilot test that a tool you planned to use won't work with your population, so you have to drop that instrument. You can't get a large enough sample by taking every third patient who meets the study criteria so you have to take all comers or relax the criteria. The secretary or physician who promised to hand out your questionnaires forgot to do so, or . . . insert your own example of Murphy's Law.

When the study you carried out was not precisely the study you planned, you can't use the proposal but instead must write new material to fit reality. It's tempting to use the old material along with the new—to present first what you wanted to do and then describe what you actually did—especially if you're feeling resentful about the help you didn't get or the hostility you did get that forced the changes. Resist the temptation. Don't talk about what you intended to do or tell readers why you couldn't do it unless you need to justify what you did or unless your methodological problems and alterations will be of interest to others.

In the following discussions I'll talk about each part of the methods section separately and try to point out what's essential to say, what you need to change in the material in your proposal, when you might need to explain the changes, and what to add.

Study Design

The Overview.   To provide a context for the details of your study methods, an overview or capsule description of the methods should be given either at the end of the literature review or at the beginning of the "Methods." One place is as good as the other, but don't give the description in both places. Unless there have been major changes in the study, this abstract of your methods will be the same as in the proposal (but put it in the past tense now). There are examples in Part One, pages 42–45, and here's another:

> An experimental group of obese patients with diabetes received weekly nutritional counseling, using behavior modification techniques, and weight monitoring for 12 weeks. To test the effectiveness of the counseling and reinforcement, the eating patterns and weights of these patients were compared to those of a comparison group of patients who received no intervention, at the end of the 12 weeks and at 24 and 48 weeks.

This tells readers what you did to whom in order to find out what. Sometimes you need to add a few more details to this basic information. For example, if you collected data on anxiety and depression to see if they had any relation to eating habits and weight, say so. Don't, however, get into the details of sample selection and measurement of variables; if you do, you'll repeat yourself later.

You do not need to sketch the design in the research report; that picture is more important to a reader examining your proposal than to one looking at your product.

Hypotheses and Research Questions.   In the research report, hypotheses are *introduced* in the past tense. For example, "The hypotheses were as follows:" Then the hypotheses themselves are *stated* in the future tense, just as in a proposal. But if you have only one or two hypotheses they can be written together using a combination of the past and conditional tenses, like this:

> It was hypothesized that the group of children who visited the hospital before coming in for their surgery would show significantly less pre- and post-operative anxiety and less post-operative depression than a group having no prior exposure to the hospital.

Research questions are also introduced in the past tense in a research report; then they are stated in the present tense, just as in a proposal, like this:

> The research questions were as follows:
> 1. Are recent life changes associated with the onset of depression in the elderly?
> 2. Is degree of functional ability associated with the level of depression in the elderly?

If you had research questions in addition to hypotheses, use the same format as for hypotheses. For example, if hypotheses are written using the past and conditional tenses, write the research questions in the same way:

> It was hypothesized that patients undergoing heart surgery who were taught relaxation techniques before the surgery would have less

pre- and post-operative anxiety than similar patients not taught relaxation techniques.

The study also explored the relationships between marital status and social supports and the level of pre- and post-operative anxiety. . . .

The study also looked at other factors that might be related to pre- and post-operative anxiety, including marital status and social supports.

In the real world there is considerable overlap between expectations and hypotheses. Depending on the degree of formality of your research proposal, you may not have stated your hypotheses directly but simply made your expectations clear in the overview. If you had no formal hypotheses in your proposal, you should have none in the report. For example, you might write:

To test the effectiveness of a charting workshop in improving documentation of home health care for Medicare reimbursement, home health care nurses in North Carolina were randomly assigned to a workshop group and a group receiving no instruction in charting; following the workshop the percentages of claims reimbursed for the two groups were compared over a six-month period.

That statement makes it clear that you expected the intervention (the charting workshop) to be effective.

Setting and Sample

Setting. If you used the setting or settings you intended to use for your study, their description in your report will be exactly as in your proposal (see pages 55–58). If you used another setting in addition to the one planned, explain why and add a description of the new setting. If you used another setting *instead of* the one planned, substitute the new description for the old one but don't tell readers there was a change in plans unless you think it will interest them.

For example, if you intended to interview patients in a physician's office and could not work out a schedule for the interviews, so switched to another, similar physician's office, you don't need to explain that change because nothing about it is important. But if you found that a particular type of setting was unworkable for your study, so you switched to a different type—say, from a private physician's office to a hospital outpatient clinic—the change needs to be explained, not only because it might have some bearing on your findings but also because it might be useful for readers to know about the problem that necessitated the change.

Describe the setting in the present tense because the setting continues to exist though your research is finished. For example, you might write:

> The study was conducted in six outpatient hemodialysis units in Iowa, Missouri, and Kansas. Two of these units serve metropolitan areas and the others serve predominantly rural areas. The metropolitan units see approximately 60 patients a week; in the rural units, the average is 40 per week.

You can omit statements about the number of people normally seen in that setting if you obtained all the subjects you needed there, but if your sample was disappointingly small, leave that information in the description, as in the example above. It helps to explain why you expected more subjects than you got.

Sample.   If you selected the sample in the manner planned, made no alterations in the criteria for inclusion in the study, and the sample turned out to be the size expected, consider yourself blessed. You can describe the sample almost exactly as you did in the proposal: first the method of selection, then the criteria for inclusion in the sample, and finally the method of assigning subjects to groups, if you had groups. Recast the description in the past tense and move on to the intervention, if applicable, or to data collection tools, saving the description of sample characteristics for "Findings."

Often, however, the setting does not produce the numbers of subjects expected. For one reason or another the patients do not appear or, perversely, they fail to meet the study criteria, or their physician refuses to give you permission to approach them, or they don't want to participate; you can probably list even more ways that plans can go awry. If your setting did not produce the sample you needed within the time you could give to the research, you must decide whether and how much to explain.

If you made no changes to deal with the disappointing sample, you can save the facts about sample size until the opening paragraph of "Findings." Just give the method of selection and the study criteria here, then move on. But the greater the discrepancy between what you hoped for and what you got, the more useful it is to tell readers about your disappointment now. Give the approximate size sample expected and the bases for your expectation (much of that was probably in the proposal and can be lifted from there), then list the reasons why the expected numbers did not materialize. Don't whine, however. The only way to deal with a problem like this is to be matter-of-fact.

If you took steps to enlarge the sample, describe them. They are usually of five types: you extended the time, did follow-up calls or mailings, added settings, altered the method of selection of part or all of the sample, or altered the criteria for inclusion in the study. (Although some of these changes may affect the generalizability of your findings, wait and discuss that issue with the findings affected.)

A time extension doesn't require any change in your description of the sample. Simply conclude by saying something like this:

> Although the expected sample was 60, only 15 subjects had been enrolled by the end of the study period because most of those eligible were too debilitated to participate. The study was therefore extended by three months and 10 more subjects were added, making a total of 25.

Follow-up efforts and their results are similarly described.

If you added an extra setting to acquire more subjects, you'll have said that already in the description of your study settings. Here, after mentioning your inability to get the sample of 60 you wanted, point out that,

> As noted above, an additional setting was used in an effort to recruit more subjects; with this setting the total sample came to 30.

If you altered the method of selection or relaxed the study criteria to acquire more subjects, you need to explain. The extent of explanation necessary depends on how far you departed from the rigor you originally intended and how well the new method succeeded in bringing in the numbers. For example, if probability sampling was the most logical way to get your sample but you gave up on it because it did not produce enough subjects or was too expensive, readers need to know that. Otherwise they may think you didn't know enough to try probability sampling.

If the new method was as good as the original and was successful in getting the sample you needed, there's no point in mentioning the change. Describe the new method as if it had been your intent to use it all along. If the new method still didn't produce enough subjects, however, you need to mention your original intent and the change you made; that's part of convincing readers you did all you could.

If you relaxed your criteria for inclusion in the study and you think readers might wonder why the criteria weren't stricter, explain. If you still didn't get enough subjects even with the liberalized criteria, explain that as well. If some of the sample members were selected using one set of criteria and the rest using another set, be sure to point out that the two groups were analyzed separately.

Conclude your description of the sample by telling how you assigned subjects to groups, if you had groups. Again, describe what you actually did; if that wasn't what you intended to do, you must decide whether and how much to explain.

Sometimes it is appropriate to conclude this section by describing the sample characteristics (instead of saving that information for "Findings"). For example, if you give the final sample size here, it seems logical to also give the sample characteristics. Also, you may find that in discussing your method of selecting the sample or assigning people to groups you must describe some of their characteristics. It is logical then to describe the rest of the characteristics here also. Or you may have acquired a very skewed sample, and discussion of efforts to correct that may require description of the skewed characteristics. In that case, too, it is wise to give the full description here. Use your judgment to decide what is the logical approach. (See pages 99–101 for suggestions on how to describe the sample.)

Intervention

If your study included an intervention, describe it step by step, giving enough detail so readers could carry out the program. But if the detail is overwhelming, include only the essentials here and save the full protocol for an appendix. Often you can lift the description of the intervention from your proposal and simply make whatever changes are needed to turn a plan into a history. If you piloted the intervention to test its feasibility for implementation, tell readers about the pilot after describing the program; if you made changes on the basis of the pilot test, indicate what they were.

Don't describe plans you couldn't carry out, unless the information is important; sometimes it *is*. For example, if you replicated a study of a procedure and found that the procedure had to be modified to be broadly usable, it is important to explain why and how, because that information might save another person pain or failure. Problems usually aren't worth mentioning, however, if they're unlikely to occur to others. Trust your judgment here; usually you'll know which problems are peculiar to your situation and which are broadly generalizable.

Be sure to put this whole section on the intervention into the past tense.

Measurement of Variables

Data Collection Instruments.   In an introductory paragraph tie each instrument securely to a variable and then describe the instruments in this order: first, physiological measures; then, scheduled observations; and, finally, questionnaires or interviews. If you used two or more measures of the same type — two questionnaires or scales, for example — describe first the tool that produced the most important findings, and follow that same order when you describe the findings. Discuss collection of demographic data last, even if you collected these first.

Generally the description of each measurement is quite similar to that in the proposal. First explain the measure, then tell how it was administered, and conclude with information on validity and reliability or pilot testing.

To make a good fit between methods and findings, there should be something in the description of your tools to explain how you collected every piece of data you will present in "Findings." For example, suppose you asked patients in a rehabilitation center to tell you their reactions to three different methods of mobilizing them. You found that the patients greatly disliked certain aspects of one method and felt so-so about the other two. In "Findings" you will doubtless elaborate on those aspects of the one method that patients disliked. In describing your questionnaire or interview, then, tell readers you asked about those aspects or otherwise show how you elicited the information, to prepare readers for the information in "Findings."

You should not describe questions or give details about measurements here if their results will not be mentioned in "Findings." For example, if you'll only briefly summarize the data from one section of your questionnaire because the six questions it contained produced little of interest, don't describe all six questions separately in "Methods" or the reader will wonder later why you give no answers to them. (Complete measurement protocols and copies of all scales, questionnaires, and interview schedules must be included in an appendix.)

The only data you do not need to prepare for in "Methods" are anecdotal data, but if you kept a log or notebook in which you jotted down patient comments or unplanned observations of your own, it is useful to report that.

Other people's instruments are described in the present tense since they are presumed to be standard and ongoing even though your study is complete, but a tool you developed is usually described in the past tense. The rest of this section on data collection tools is also in the past.

Validity and Reliability.   Conclude the description of each tool with information on validity and reliability or pilot testing. If you used instruments developed by others, you generally do not need to discuss the means used to establish the validity and reliability of the tools. Those details were needed in your proposal to convince readers that the tools would work for you. Either the tools worked for you or they didn't, regardless of the thoroughness used by others to establish validity and reliability. So cut out the details; simply note whether validity and reliability were established and reference your statements so interested readers can check them. If, however, you plan to focus later on a tool's shortcomings, modifications, or refinements, you need to include the details as preparation for the comments you'll make in your findings or discussion section.

If the tools you used were your own, include all the information on pilot tests or tool revisions or efforts to establish validity and reliability, since these will affect the credibility of your findings.

Changes in Plans or Organization. If you had to abandon a measurement in mid-study, omit all mention of it unless you want to focus on problems with the tool later, or unless you want to present the data you collected before you let the tool go. (If you use data collected with this tool, you must indicate how you kept those subjects measured with the tool separate from those not measured.)

Sometimes you have to alter your data collection plans substantially, and this may be important to tell readers. Suppose, for example, you found in a pilot test that the tools you designed or took from another investigator were unworkable or required serious revisions. You'll need to explain this fully and you may also need to alter the organization of your data collection section. Try this order: first briefly introduce your tools, next introduce the pilot test, and then discuss the testing and resulting revisions as you describe each tool.

Your outline would look like this:

Measurement of Variables

1. Introduction to variables measured and tools used to measure them
2. Pilot testing and tool revision
   a. Introduction
   b. For each tool pilot tested,

(1) brief description of original tool
(2) results of pilot test
(3) consequent revisions
(4) description of the tool as used in the study

If you used a pilot test as a basis for developing a questionnaire or observation checklist, try a similar organization; first describe the pilot test, then the resulting tool. Suppose, for example, you developed and tested a questionnaire to elicit information about the concerns of family members of patients in intensive care units. You began with a pilot test in which you asked a number of such family members open-ended questions about their concerns. You then categorized and coded the answers and, on the basis of commonalities in the responses, developed a checklist of concerns as the heart of your questionnaire. Clearly the pilot test should be discussed before the checklist. Always let the logic of the work dictate your organization.

Research Procedures

Your research procedures should be described chronologically, like a story. First tell how you acquired subjects and then what you did with them. Omit the details on how you gained access to the subjects. In the proposal those details were needed to persuade readers that you could indeed acquire a sample. Now they are superfluous. Include only the information about gaining access that might be important for others. For example, if you made extra efforts to ingratiate yourself with supervisors whose staff nurses you wished to observe and as a consequence your path was smoothed, it is helpful to pass on such information so that others can try the same tactics. But unless your means of proceeding stand out like that, omit them. Also omit all names. Simply indicate by title who gave you permission to conduct the study and then tell how you approached potential subjects.

Also, don't tell readers how you explained the study, gained consent from subjects, and assured confidentiality and anonymity; like the nuts and bolts of gaining access, this information is important in a proposal and unnecessary in a report. Simply point out that all subjects signed a consent form and that confidentiality and anonymity were assured. If the data were not kept confidential and anonymous, explain. Sample copies of the information you gave subjects and the consent form should be included in the appendix.

Include all the details of your research procedures that will be important for your findings. For studies with an intervention, this part of the story is usually a clear series of events: first a pretest or series of pre-treatment measurements, then a treatment, then post-treatment measurements, and sometimes later follow-up. If you had both an experimental and a comparison group, first tell the story for the experimental group, then for the comparison group.

If your study included no intervention, simply describe the procedure for collecting data. For example, if you mailed out a questionnaire in September, did one follow-up mailing in November, and made a further follow-up phone call in January, tell readers the schedule.

Usually the procedure section is very close to that in the proposal, minus the details that are no longer needed. If you did not follow the procedure you planned, describe what you actually did, not what you planned to do, and don't discuss the changes unless they are important for explaining your findings or of interest in themselves.

Never describe the intervention or data collection tools in this section. Here you tell where, when, and to whom something was done; the what, why, and how have already been explained. If you find you're beginning to explain those again, look back at the earlier sections of "Methods," compare, and cut out the overlaps.

Unless you have given dates in describing the steps in your research procedure, conclude this section by giving the time frame of the study—May to November, say.

Chapter 9

Findings

With a wheelbarrow full of data and computer printout piling up on the floor, it's often hard to know where or how to begin reporting your findings. Never write straight from the computer printout; if you do, your findings will look like undigested bits of this and that.

To begin, group your data, make up basic tables, and get on paper some notes about the findings that strike you as important. Then organize your data using the outline below. Writing from tables and notes will make it easier to summarize and highlight.

Findings

A. Introduction

B. Description of the sample
   1. Size of final sample and explanations for losses during the study
   2. Sample characteristics
   3. Differences between groups

C. Major findings

1. Scores or measurements of the variables of interest and differences between groups, if applicable
2. Secondary, less important, or itemized findings

D. Hypothesis testing, if applicable
   1. Maneuvers to make the data more amenable to testing
   2. Results of hypothesis testing

E. Additional analyses or findings

While it isn't absolutely necessary, it is often helpful, depending on the complexity of the findings, to begin with an introductory paragraph that tells readers what this section contains and how it is organized. The more varied your data, the more important it is to give readers a guide to their presentation.

Sample Characteristics

Describe the sample at the beginning of "Findings" unless you described it in the methods section. Give its potential size, then its actual size, or its size at the beginning and end of the study. For example, if you mailed out 1,500 questionnaires of which 100 were not deliverable and 750 were returned, give all three figures, in that order. And if 14 of the 750 were unusable, explain why and give the final tally. Similarly, if you gave a pretest to 60 patients, taught all 60 about their medication and then gave each of them a posttest, but could only get 33 to come back and complete a follow-up posttest two months later, give all the figures. If you lost subjects along the way, explain why, and if your subjects were assigned to different groups, give the losses by groups.

After presenting the numbers, highlight the important characteristics of the sample—all the factors you collected data on because you thought they might affect the findings. These characteristics may be of several types: demographic (age, race, sex), social and economic (occupation, education, socioeconomic status, marital status), lifestyle (diet, smoking, exercise), genetic or biological characteristics associated with disease, or even the incidence or prevalence of disease. Begin your description with the demographics, and move from these basic characteristics to those which are more particular. Don't mix up characteristics of different types — that is, don't give age, then education, then sex. Give age and sex together, then move on to education. Grouping characteristics in this manner makes it easier for readers to grasp a lot of information quickly.

First characterize the sample as a whole, then present any differences between groups and indicate whether or not the differences were statistically significant, giving the relevant statistics in parentheses. Don't run through the whole list of characteristics for both groups; just point out differences that were sizable or significant. Remember that the only reason you do this is to let readers know there are group differences that might make a difference in the validity of the findings.

Describe the sample in general terms; don't choke readers with a mass of figures. In a research report, unlike an article, you have all the room you want. So depict the sample fully in a table or tables; then look at each table, see what it shows, put it away, and give only the highlights in the text, using approximate words like "a few," "a third," "nearly half," "the majority," "most," "three quarters," "the great majority," "nearly all." Give percentages or numbers in parentheses, thus:

> Most of the subjects were under 30 (78%), white (69%) females (63%). About half (48%) were college graduates and nearly all (90%) were employed full-time.

If you write from memory instead of directly from the table, you'll be more likely to give the kind of summary description readers want. Then pick the precise percentages or numbers out of the table and insert them. Refer readers to the table for details.

In discussing the sample and in presenting findings, use percentages if the sample is large, but use numbers if it is small. It is ludicrous to say "33% of the sample" when you are talking about three people. And it makes readers think you're trying to put one over on them. In his delightful book, *How to Write and Publish a Scientific Paper*, Robert A. Day quotes the former editor-in-chief of *Infection and Immunology* to bring home the point: "33⅓% of the mice used in this experiment were cured by the test drug; 33⅓% of the test population were unaffected by the drug and remained in a moribund condition; the third mouse got away" (p. 35).

If you have 15 or 20 people, it's wise to use both numbers and percentages. It is particularly helpful to give both when you have a small sample with groups of unequal sizes; the percentages allow comparisons of unequal groups while the numbers keep the reader firmly planted in reality. Suppose, for example, that in your sample of 25 patients with diabetes, 11 were female and 14 male. You might want readers to know that "Seven of the females (64%) and four of the males (39%) were obese." By saying it this way you allow the reader to see both the small difference in numbers and the large difference in percentages.

The Data

Put aside for a moment the statistical maneuvers you've been struggling with and describe the data. Tell readers the results of your measurements, the outcomes of your observations, the answers to the questions you asked.

If your study was designed to test the effectiveness of an intervention, present the figures that show whether the treatment was effective. Let's say you used the number of pain medications taken by patients over a week's time, before and after relaxation training, to judge the effectiveness of relaxation in reducing chronic pain. You not only compared the experimental patients to themselves but also to a group receiving no training. First tell how many pain medications the experimental and comparison group patients were taking before the training, then tell how many the experimental group took afterwards, and how many the comparison group took during the same period.

After you have presented the pre- and post-scores, give the change in scores; then note the differences between pre-, post-, and change in scores and conclude by indicating whether or not these differences were statistically significant, with the significance figures in parentheses, e.g., "($p < 0.05$)." (More about significance later.)

If you used several measures to test the effectiveness of the intervention, present the findings in the order in which you described your measurement tools in the methods section. First come physiological measures, then scheduled observations, and finally questionnaires or interviews. (If some of these measurements showed significant differences and some did not, you might want to alter the order so that you present the data on significant differences first. Be sure then to comment on the inconsistency of your measurements.) Fit anecdotal data in wherever they are useful.

If your study included no intervention, present the most important findings first. Usually that is the information needed to test your hypotheses or research questions. If you had more than one hypothesis or research question, don't automatically present your data in the order that you listed the hypotheses or questions in the "Methods" section. Instead, present what's most important or striking first, and reorder your arrangement of hypotheses or questions in "Methods" to correspond.

Sometimes your hypotheses were not supported but you made other interesting and important discoveries. In that case, quickly present the data on the original hypotheses, note that your expectations were not met, and move on to what matters.

In describing data, first give information for the sample as a whole; then, if you had groups or subsamples, present the data for the groups separately. Point out, for example, that the mean score on the depression scale was high for the sample as a whole, and give the figures. Then give the scores for the subsample who were drug users and the subsample who were not, and indicate which subgroup mean was higher and which lower, both absolutely and in relation to the total group. Or point out that your sample of diabetic patients scored low on a test of their knowledge of good nutritional principles, and then give the scores for the subsample who were overweight and the subsample who were not.

When you present mean scores or rankings, it is helpful to indicate the range of responses or standard deviation. Depending on the number and complexity of your measurements you may also need to remind readers of the possible range on the instrument, even though you have already presented that information in "Methods." Similarly, you may need to repeat the norm.

Give the data on each of your major variables before you examine the significance of differences between subsamples or groups. Remember, tests of significance have no meaning for readers until the differences being tested are made plain. Deal with correlations as with differences. First give the figures, then the correlation, and finally the significance, or lack of it, with statistics in parentheses, e.g., "($r=0.2735$, $p<.05$)."

Tables and Figures

Presenting information can be tricky; often there's a lot of it, and since a report is supposed to be complete you have to find a way to say it all. But some of it is complex and hard to shape into sentences. Tables are a big help here. In a report you can use as many as you need since you have unlimited space. Construct a table whenever you have repeated numbers that will be hard to group or grasp in the narrative. The more figures you need to present in order to make a point or convey a clear sense of the data, the more you need a table to help readers see the patterns in the data. If you can easily present the information in words, a table is pointless.

Although you can have all the tables you want, whenever possible try to condense your information and combine tables, making two or three into one. A good rule of thumb is this: If two different tables have one or more columns that are the same, try combining them. This will bring you closer to an article, where space is tight and expensive and tables have to be limited.

Never present the same information in both a table and the narrative. A table gives a comprehensive and detailed view; the narrative should highlight the table, presenting the main points to be gleaned from it. The table can then serve the reader as a reference while the narrative moves on. The narrative should be clear without requiring reference to tables and, conversely, tables should be understandable without the narrative. This means that the title of a table should make it obvious what the table is about. Headings should be concise but clearly indicate how the data are organized. Similar elements should be read down, not across, and totals generally come at the bottom.

Include no tables that you don't refer to in the narrative, and refer to them in parentheses instead of dragging them into the sentence. For example, don't write, "Table 5 shows that the knowledge scores of all but five patients improved." Instead say, "The knowledge scores of all but five patients improved (see Table 5)." The reference in the text must always precede the table.

Graphs and charts convey information more dramatically than tables, and sometimes more clearly. Consider using them whenever you want to represent patterns and proportions. But don't give both tables and figures setting forth the same information.

The APA style manual gives detailed suggestions for constructing both tables and figures, of all types.

Presenting the Information

The computer printout doesn't help to shape your findings into sentences and while a table helps you decide what needs to be said in the narrative, it won't help with the words. The basic rule is this: make sure words say what you mean them to. That sounds elementary but it's not always easy; read every sentence aloud to check. Here are a few suggestions.

Distinguish carefully between *majority* and *most*. The first means anything over half, but the latter generally requires at least two-thirds and is better with three-quarters. You can use "a sizable majority" to cover the territory in between. For example, you might write:

> Most of the patients (83%) rated their pain as moderate or severe. A sizable majority (65%) also scored high on the first portion of the anxiety inventory. Somewhat fewer though still a majority (52%) scored high on the second portion.

Be sure you're describing the right difference. If you mean to say a larger percentage of the RNs than of the NAs were married, don't say more RNs than NAs were married. Proportions and numbers aren't equivalent.

Don't confuse *probability* and *reality*. If in your sample a larger percentage of the men than of the women were alcohol abusers, say so. If your sampling procedure warrants, you may be able to conclude that men are more likely than women to abuse alcohol. But don't say, "In this sample men were more likely than women to be alcohol abusers." They either drank too much or they didn't; probability, as represented by "likely," doesn't enter into it. Only in reporting a complex regression analysis does it make sense to talk about risk and probability in the sample you studied.

Don't confuse a *pattern* with a *trend*. A pattern can be seen when differences existing at one time are consistent among different groups. For example, you may see a pattern in the differences between male and female scores on depression scales in all the age groups in your sample. In contrast, a trend involves change in a consistent direction over time; you might see a trend toward healthier lifestyles among the middle and upper-middle socio-economic groups in the last decade but no similar trend among lower income groups.

Words like *increase* and *decrease* always involve change, while *more* and *less*, *higher* and *lower*, can indicate difference *or* change. Thus, if you assessed mobility once in two groups of elderly patients and found that those who exercised regularly could walk farther and more easily than those who did not exercise, you can't say "mobility was increased" in those who exercised, you must say they were "more mobile." But if you assessed mobility in a group, then had them exercise regularly for a month and afterwards assessed mobility again, you can say their mobility "increased" or they were "more mobile" after the exercise program.

Complete your comparisons. If you say the experimental subjects were more relaxed or less anxious, don't just leave them hanging there; indicate whom or to what you are comparing them. Were they less anxious than another group? Than themselves before or after exercise? Than the sample in another study? Than the general population?

Be careful to use the right sets of words for your comparisons. Here are some samples:

more	*or* less	→ than
higher	*or* lower	→ than
similar		→ to
as well	*or* as poorly	→ as
as high	*or* as low	→ as

| different | → from |
| differ | → from |

For example, you might write:

On the posttest the group who had exercised regularly had *lower* anxiety scores *than* the group who had not exercised.

On the pretest the experimental group scores were *similar to* those of the comparison group.

Subjects who were not taught about insulin administration did *as well* on the test *as* those who had been taught.

On the posttest the experimental group scores *differed* significantly *from* those of the control group.

Different than is always followed by a clause:

The test scores suggested different conclusions than they did a year earlier.

Don't write, "The experimental group's anxiety was higher as compared to the control group." The phrase *as compared to* takes the form *high*, not *higher*. If you are careful to distinguish words like *more* and *less* from words like *increase* and *decrease*, you will surely not stray into swampy constructions like "On the posttest the anxiety level of the experimental group was increased when compared to the control group."

Watch out for words that are easily confused—*ratings* and *scores*, for example. A subject may *score* well or poorly on a test of knowledge but he or she *rates* the severity of pain or the importance of salary on a scale. Thus you should refer to *pain ratings*, not *pain scores*, and *ratings* or *rankings* of importance (but not *importance scores*).

Comprise and *compose* are trickier. *Comprise* is the parts forming the whole; *compose* is the whole formed by parts. Thus, "the group *comprised* five members, all of whom suffered toxic side effects from methadone," but "the group was *composed* of those five people."

To say a group was *composed* of 15 people with lung cancer indicates that those 15 people made up the whole group, but *in-*

clude can refer to some or all. For example, if you write, "The experimental group included 15 patients with lung cancer," you may be telling readers that there were 15 patients in the experimental group, all with lung cancer, but the sentence may also mean that among the patients in the experimental group, 15 had lung cancer. Say what you mean.

When you discuss a question or statement on a questionnaire or scale, describe it clearly the first time you mention it and then give it a tag or label to save space. Don't refer to "Question 1" or "Question 2," for this requires readers to remember the trivial or look back to discover what you're talking about. And don't refer to questions or statements as "items" just because that's what they are on the computer printout.

Present all your findings in the past tense, and don't lead into them with wordy introductions. For example, don't write:

> The results of this study demonstrated that intracranial pressure decreased in patients whose families provided soothing stimuli.

Go straight to the point: "Intracranial pressure decreased. . . ."

Don't tell readers how interesting or important the findings were. Show them. In other words, don't introduce a finding with, "It was particularly interesting to note that. . . ." If the finding was striking and you don't think readers will see that, explain. At most, cue them with a word. For example, you might write,

> Interestingly, charting on the unit was more complete during the study period than before it, even though recordkeeping was not a focus of the investigation.

That one word *interestingly* is enough to alert readers to your sense that there was something out of the ordinary about this finding.

Never begin a sentence with numerals. If it's awkward to write out a number like "five hundred eighty-seven," revise your sentence so you don't begin with the number. For instance, you could write "A total of 587. . . ." There's more than one way to skin a cat!

Try to vary your sentence constructions. Nothing is more deadly than endless repetitions of a formula such as "Eight percent said they liked it, 18% said they disliked it, 28% said they didn't care, 38% said they hadn't thought about it, 48% said they didn't know what it was," and on and on and on. Don't vary your sentences, however, by writing them backward: "Of particular importance was the staff's awareness that they were involved in research." You wouldn't talk like that, so try to avoid writing that way.

One way to vary your constructions is to read well-written articles in a journal you respect, copy the sentences you like, and try the same constructions to report your own findings. It is also helpful to write from memory rather than straight from a table (or worse, printout). Look at the table whose data you want to highlight, then put it away and recite the important information aloud to yourself. You'll doubtless say it clearly when you speak it; transfer the words to paper before they get bent out of shape by the desire to write scholarly prose. Then look back at the table to check your accuracy.

Significance is a troublesome word, but in a useful book called *Statistics Without Tears*, Derek Rowntree does much to demystify it. All the word means, says Rowntree, is *real*. A difference that's statistically significant is one you can count on to exist. It may not be an interesting or important difference, but you can be pretty sure it didn't appear by chance. In the same way, a correlation that is statistically significant is one that's almost surely real, though whether the size of it is enough to matter is another question.

Report significance tests after reporting differences. And in reporting these tests, name them but don't describe them or tell why you picked them. You need to explain a test only when it is not standard and you need to tell why you used a test only when it is not generally considered appropriate for your data. (In the latter case you must not only tell readers why you thought this test would work, but you must also explain why some other test that might seem more appropriate would not work.)

Never name the statistical package you used to prepare the data for testing or describe your other technical operations. That preparation is like your work in the library: you have to do a lot more of it than you can write about. Readers don't need the information and it is an intrusion in the report. If you indicate what test you used and what confidence level you set, they'll understand the rest.

When you describe significance testing, the p level is generally given in parentheses and p is written in lower case and italicized.

When your differences or correlations were not statistically significant, do not moan pitifully to readers that they were "almost significant" or "almost reached significance" or "showed a trend toward significance." There's no such thing as a trend toward significance; differences either are significant or they aren't. If you found a difference that was big enough to seem important to you but was not statistically significant, and you think that might be because the sample was small, it's sensible to point that out. Similarly, if your sample was big and the difference was small, albeit significant, you need to point out that the significance may have been merely a function of sample size. That knife cuts both ways.

Remember that a finding—i.e., a fact—is never statistically significant. Only relationships—differences or associations—are statistically significant.

Hypothesis Testing

The most logical way to let readers know whether or not your data supported your hypothesis is to present the data, note the difference or correlation, indicate whether or not it was significant, and conclude that the hypothesis was or was not supported. This organization is easiest to follow when your study included an intervention and you had only one measure of its effectiveness—say, difference in number of postoperative complications—or a couple of complementary measures like reported pain and scores on a depression scale pre- and post-intervention.

It's more complicated when you have a pile of data and a string of hypotheses on related but nonetheless different variables. In that case it's best to present all the data first and then deal with all the hypotheses in a separate section in the same order that you presented the data.

Don't refer to hypotheses simply by number, making readers look elsewhere to figure out what is Hypothesis #1 and what is #2. And don't just dump the hypotheses out on the page as if they had nothing to do with your narrative. Introduce them, thus: "The first hypothesis was as follows" or, better still, "It was hypothesized that . . . ." (Remember in this latter construction that you must use the past and conditional tenses: "It was hypothesized that children who experienced the death of a sibling would show more anxiety than children without siblings.") If a particular hypothesis was not supported, you can lead into that by saying, "While it was hypothesized that . . .," and conclude, "the data showed no significant differences and thus did not support the hypothesis."

Exploratory Analyses

After you've dealt with your hypotheses, describe any additional or exploratory analyses you undertook and present the findings. Introduce each analysis by indicating its purpose or by giving a rationale for doing it. Next describe the scope of the analysis and any maneuvers you made with the data in order to do the analysis (such as collapsing categories or developing a scale); then present the findings. Sometimes these are the most interesting findings in the study; don't fail to give readers the interesting information just because you weren't originally looking for it.

Anecdotal Data

Some people save their anecdotal data for the "Discussion," but unscheduled or chance observations, comments by patients or staff or families, and other anecdotal data are part of your findings and are better put in this section. They have two major functions. If you found what you were looking for, anecdotal data confirm your numbers and make them come alive; if the results were not what you hoped for, they help explain why. (In fact, unsystematic data of this sort are often extremely suggestive and may point the way to new studies that take into account aspects of the problem that were not recognized earlier.) The more specific and concrete the information, the more interesting and useful it is. If you have so much anecdotal data that you have to summarize it, be sure to use the most interesting comments to highlight the group data.

Comments

Sometimes it's hard to decide what kind of comments are appropriate in "Findings" and what should be saved for "Discussion." The general rule is this: Comment on particular findings as you present them, then discuss the overall meanings of your study after you've presented all the particular findings.

If a study produced only two or three major pieces of information, there's no need to discuss them in "Findings"; save the comments for the "Discussion." But if you have more than a very few pieces of data, comment as you go. Otherwise there'll be so many comments in the discussion section that the reader won't be able to remember what information all those comments are based on, and you'll have to repeat a lot of your findings to make the comments understandable.

Your comments should answer questions like these: What does it matter if a difference was statistically significant? Does it mean that your intervention was probably effective, or could the difference have resulted from another cause? Was the difference large enough to make a difference in the real world of patient care? If the difference was not significant, was it still large enough to be important? Does it warrant further investigation? Why was it not larger?

Don't make comments that simply repeat your data. For example, if you found that the depression levels of elderly women in your sample were significantly higher than those of elderly men, don't point out that this indicates the elderly women in your sample were more depressed than the men. A comment should elaborate on or explain the data, not repeat it in other words.

In commenting, watch your language. If the findings are strong, they may "demonstrate" or "show" that a particular intervention improves patient outcomes. If they are more tentative, use words like *indicate* or *suggest*. Remember that research never "proves" anything, and variation is "explained" by, not "caused" by, for correlation is not cause.

Use expressions like "it seems" and "it appears" judiciously, and avoid "it would seem," "it would appear" and "I feel"—or worse, "it is felt by this investigator." In most cases those expressions are a way of saying to the reader, "I might be wrong and I want you to know that I know it." If your comments and conclusions are of necessity tentative, those distancing phrases will help protect you, but avoid the temptation to be overly self-protective. If the evidence is insufficient or open to question and you are presenting merely "suggestive findings," say so explicitly. Don't use qualifiers like *seems* as a substitute for articulating your evidence. If you have reason to conclude that physicians are largely responsible for the operating-room delays you've observed, lay out the evidence. Don't leave what you know unsaid and shrink back from the point, trying to cover your vulnerability with "seems."

If there were differences between the groups in your sample, comment on their possible effects as you present the findings that may have been affected. For example, if one group of surgery patients was significantly older than the other, readers need to be told that age might have affected outcomes. If the differences had no impact make that clear as well.

If shortcomings in the data collection tools appear to have affected particular findings, point that out also as you present the findings. And if you want to compare particular findings to those of other investigators, this is a good place to do so. More general comparisons with other studies should be saved for your discussion.

Sometimes you'll find that the problem is not what you thought it was, is bigger than you knew, exists other than where you expected, cannot be solved, or is unlikely to be solved unless something else happens. Present the evidence as the conclusion to your findings, which will lead readers into the discussion.

References

Day, R.A. (1983). *How to write and publish a scientific paper* (2nd ed.). Philadelphia: ISI Press.

Rowntree, D. (1982). *Statistics without tears: A primer for non-mathematicians.* New York: Scribner.

Chapter 10

Discussion

Thinking Through

The "Discussion" is the hardest section of a report to write, both because it requires more thinking than any other part and because it's the last to be done. Most researchers are pretty weary by the time they get to the end of a study, and those finishing degree requirements or coming to the close of a grant period are often pressed for time. That combination makes it hard to enjoy mulling over findings to squeeze out all their meanings. Hard as it may be, however, it is important to think through the "Discussion" section; you'll have to do that for an article and the further you take the process now, the easier it will be to go the rest of the way later.

This section should answer the question, "So what?" Ask yourself: So what if nurses exposed to cancer chemotherapy drugs show no immediate physiological consequences? So what if patients in a rural clinic are more satisfied with nurse practitioner care than with physician care? So what if the major reasons nurses give for leaving the ICU are job stress and lack of administrative support? In short, what do your research findings amount to? What can they mean for others? What difference do they make?

Jot down your ideas as they come to you, without worrying

about organization. That will come later. For now you need meaning, not order. You can make good use of thesis or dissertation committee members to help you figure out what it all means; give them a draft of the findings and ask for a meeting at which you'll present your initial conclusions and get them to brainstorm further with you. It's much easier to get people's ideas in a conversation than in writing; the latter takes more time and effort than most people have to spare. But it's a good idea to tape the conversation or at least take notes. Use your friends and colleagues to help you think through your conclusions also. Anybody with a clear head will see interesting ideas and questions in the material.

Organization

The "Discussion" has four basic parts:

A. Brief summary of the major findings
B. Overall meaning of the findings (relationships shown, generalizations to be made)
C. Limitations to generalizability
D. Implications for research, theory, and practice

To begin, briefly summarize the findings. Obviously, the more numerous and complex the findings, the longer the summary. But the purpose is to lead readers into a discussion, not to repeat what you have just said. So be as brief as possible. A paragraph, two at most, should suffice. Summarize the findings in the order you presented them, putting the most important first. Avoid details and don't try to be complete, just give highlights.

Next, tell readers what the findings mean. Do not repeat the comments made earlier; discuss overall meanings. What can the data, considered together, tell readers about the question you set out to answer, the problem you tried to solve, or the theoretical proposition you tested? Do your data provide a clear answer or solution? If not, do you have a partial answer, or do your data lead to further questions? Do you have some unexpected conclusions to offer on the matter or on a related issue?

This is the place to advance a claim about the importance of your findings and compare your conclusions with those of other investigators. For example, if your evidence indicates that nursing home staff's attitudes toward the elderly are positively affected by continuing education, you'll want to emphasize that and say whether and how this confirms or differs from the conclusions of other investigators. If no comparisons come naturally, however, don't force them. Your findings can be important without having much to do with what others have found.

After you advance the claim for the importance of what you've discovered, you must back away, qualify, admit to limitations. But suppress the urge to recite a litany of the imperfections of your study; instead, discuss shortcomings as they limit the credibility, generalizability, or usefulness of the findings. For example, if your sample of rural clinic patients who preferred nurse practitioner care to physician care was a sample of convenience, don't say "Alas" and stop there. Tell readers how this might affect the credibility of your finding that the people preferred nurses.

When you raise questions about credibility or caution readers about generalizing your findings, respond to any of the questions or qualifications you can. For example, let's say you used a convenience sample to evaluate home care for terminally ill cancer patients in a rural Southern town. After presenting patients' and families' positive reports of the quality of the final days, you must point to the limited generalizability of these data. Then, however, you should remind readers that it would be unrealistic to expect any other kind of sample and note the strengths of your data, concluding with a discussion of ways they can be shored up— perhaps by a replication of the study in another area of the country, using a population with different diseases and patient characteristics.

The discussion of limitations thus leads straight to suggestions for further research, but don't suggest more study if it's unnecessary or likely to be unproductive. In particular, don't suggest a replication of your own study unless your findings are really in need of further verification. Never suggest something so vague as "further research in this area." Any questions or problems for further study should be specific, and the discussion should make clear their importance and the feasibility of studying them.

The discussion of unresolved problems or unanswered questions is another place where you might compare your findings and conclusions to those of others. Comparisons here can reinforce a statement that further study is needed or indicate different directions for study.

To conclude the "Discussion" section, emphasize the importance of the study findings *now*. The final paragraphs should be strong and positive. Present the implications of the findings for theory and conclude with implications for practice. Point out the effectiveness and feasibility of the intervention and suggest how it may best be used in other settings, or tell readers what interventions are suggested by the data, what nurses and others need to do, and how they can go about it. Don't preach or moralize, however. Let your persuasive presentation of facts and ideas lead readers to put your findings into their practice.

Dealing With Disappointment

If you found neither what you hoped for nor anything else satisfactory, use the "Discussion" section to explain. Don't flinch from your findings. Begin by summarizing them clearly and telling readers the conclusions they point to. If those conclusions are not what you'd like them to be, you have to do some hard thinking and decide whether you are convinced by the data. If you are, discuss what you found in the same positive tone you'd take had you found what you expected. Explain why you found the unexpected: Was it impossible to foresee the depth or scope of the problem? Was the problem other than anyone thought? Are the reported studies from a different era and a different way of thinking, such that they were misleading? Does the theory you based your study on need reexamination?

The fact that you are convinced by the data probably means you don't think the unexpected findings resulted from flaws in your research, so the explanations should not include a list of your mistakes or bad luck. Instead, give readers a sense of how the views of this matter need to change and move thus to listing the questions that remain unanswered, the verifications still needed, the possibilities that more of the unexpected is to be expected. Conclude with the implications for practice *now*.

If you are not convinced that the data reflect reality, a major part of the explanation is probably the inadequacy of the research that produced the data. Suppose, for example, that the experimental group of students who had an orientation to the operating room scored lower on a posttest than the comparison group who received no orientation. But you still think the orientation is a useful teaching method. Why are you not convinced by your findings? Why should readers not be convinced? Did the test not reflect the information given during the orientation? Did the comparison group have other, perhaps better opportunities to get the information on the test? Were the characteristics of the experimental group such that they might have been expected to assimilate this kind of information less easily than the comparison group?

Lay out the possibilities as a prelude to suggesting further research with more appropriate methods or more rigorous controls; the more specific your suggestions, the better. Then end the discussion by pointing out that until further study is done, no clear answers can be given to the question, or no conclusions drawn about the best solution to the problem.

Sometimes people are so sure of the answers they propose that they cannot believe those answers could be wrong. Or they may be so certain that the theory they've adopted reflects reality accurately that they cannot see it won't fit the data. If your study design and procedures were flawless and you are still unconvinced by the data they produced, ask yourself why. Keep asking yourself why you don't believe what you see until you either give up your preconceptions and give in to the data, or you discover a reason for thinking them suspect.

If you don't give in, then you must show the reader why the data are unconvincing. That requires careful reasoning. It's hard to do, but you may come up with ideas for further study or new approaches to interpretation or practical suggestions for solving the problem. This kind of puzzling over the possible meanings of disappointing data, if clearly articulated, can be an exciting conclusion to your research.

PART THREE

Writing an Article Reporting
Research

Chapter 11

Organization

Research is pointless unless it's made available to others, so writing an article to report a study is as important as any other step in the research process. Alas, many people never take that final step; as a consequence, nurse researchers often tread the same ground over and over, and nursing knowledge doesn't advance as fast as it might.

Reporting your research is not as difficult as writing most other articles. For one thing, the outline for a research article is more or less fixed; you don't have to worry about how to go from beginning to end. Moreover, you already have your materials: a formal protocol for an intervention or at least some data collection tools and the findings they produced. You may well have written a proposal or both a proposal and a report of some kind, a thesis, or dissertation, so that much of the material is already on paper. The main work will then be pruning and shaping.

Below is an outline for a fairly standard research article. The parts of the article may stretch or contract, the organization may vary, and the emphasis and tone may grow more or less formal depending on the audience or journal for which you're writing. This chapter will be devoted to the basic outline and its variations. Then we'll discuss the standard research article; the one adapted from a thesis, dissertation, or report; and finally the article that is written straight from the data sheets. Throughout will be examples from published work.

The Basic Outline

All articles reporting research have four basic parts:

Why I Did It
What I Did
What I Found
What It Means

If you think of the article in this personal way, it is easier to write without being intimidated by your (and others') conceptions (often false) of what scientific writing is or should be. But think of the four parts more formally, if that works better for you, as follows:

Introduction (also called review of the literature or problem or rationale or background for the study, and sometimes left untitled)

Methods (or methods and procedures, or materials, methods and subjects)

Findings (or results)

Discussion (also called implications or conclusions)

The complete outline looks like this:

Research Article Outline

I. Introduction and review of the literature
    A. The problem (question) needing study
    B. Work already done on the problem (theoretical and empirical)

    C. Gaps or shortcomings in the work done to date

    D. The purpose of the work being reported

II. Methods

    A. Overview of the study, with hypotheses or research questions, if applicable

    B. Setting and sample

    C. Intervention, if applicable

    D. Data collection instruments

III. Findings

    A. Description of the sample

    B. Description of the data

    C. Hypothesis testing, if applicable

    D. Exploratory analyses, if applicable

IV. Discussion

    A. The major findings and their general meanings

    B. Limitations to the generalizability or usefulness of the findings

    C. Further research needed

    D. Implications for theory, if applicable

    E. Usefulness of the findings for practice

Variations in Format

The basic outline for an article reporting research is more or less followed by every journal publishing research. There are variations, however. For instance, one nursing research journal requires this format:

Unlabelled introduction

Method
    Sample/subjects
    Instruments or measures
    Procedure

Results

Discussion

In that journal, the overview of the study and the hypotheses come at the end of the introductory section, replacing a statement of purpose. The "Methods" section begins with a description of setting and sample, and research procedures are presented in a separate section at the end of "Methods" instead of being integrated into the other sections. But this is still the same basic outline as that given above. Other journals may be more flexible about formats and labels, but still want you to cover the same material.

If you check articles in nursing journals, you'll note other variations in organization. Sometimes the study purpose is given in the opening sentence of the introduction instead of at the end. And if the introduction is brief, the purpose may not be stated at all, but communicated directly or indirectly in the overview of the study methods. Sometimes the introduction and review of the literature appear under separate headings, and there may be another separate section headed "Theoretical Framework" or "Conceptual Framework." The sample characteristics may be described in "Methods" or in "Findings"; results and discussion may be separate or together; and sometimes after the "Discussion" section there is a final section called "Implications" or "Conclusions" or "Summary and Conclusions." But these are minor variations in the same basic outline.

Variations in Emphasis and Tone

Journals differ considerably in the space and emphasis given to each of the parts of an article. Roughly speaking, there are three types of nursing journals: research journals, specialty journals, and broad spectrum or general audience journals. All three publish research, but they present it quite differently. Research journals usually publish studies in all fields, with emphasis on the theoretical and methodological aspects of the work. They will publish proportionally longer literature reviews than most other journals, allow more tables and more details about tool development or types of analysis, and be more interested in the implications for further research than in long descriptions of how easily a treatment can be put into practice.

The specialty journals, appealing to nurses in a particular clinical area or to educators or administrators, usually publish research only in their area and are fairly flexible about how it is presented. They are likely to want more space given to results and their implications for practice than to methods or details of analytical procedures, and the literature review is commonly very brief. In recent years, however, many of these journals have published studies written just as they might be for a research journal.

The general interest or broad spectrum journals want fewer details about research methods, even less of a literature review, and a great deal of information about the treatment studied or the question explored and its importance for nurses in practice.

Many journals in other health and health-related fields publish studies by nurses, and their emphases also differ; some are more interested in the practical applications of research, others in theoretical or methodological aspects. As a rule, however, they expect reports of studies to be lean and do not publish long literature reviews or details of analyses unless the latter are out of the ordinary.

The tone of the writing, like the emphasis, also varies from one journal to another. Those aimed at broad audiences tend to be informal and personal, those aimed primarily at readers of research tend to be impersonal and formal. Articles for broad audiences, even articles describing research, may begin with an anecdote or human interest story to set the stage for what is to come. That would be unthinkable in a research journal. You will see "I" and "you" more frequently in journals for broad audiences, while the third person and passive voice are seen more often in research journals. You will also find some contractions ("don't") in the former, but never in the latter. If you compare journals, you will see other differences in style and tone; depending on how you write, your article will be acceptable in some places and not in others.

Two good sources of information on nursing journals and health care journals that publish writing by nurses are McCloskey and Swanson (1982), "Publishing Opportunities for Nurses: A Comparison of 100 Journals," and Swanson and McCloskey (1982), "The Manuscript Review Process of Nursing Journals." The authors categorize journals according to audience and preferred subject matter and give practical details about length, procedures for submission, the review process, and reasons for rejection.

References

McCloskey, J. C., & Swanson, E. (1982). Publishing opportunities for nurses: A comparison of 100 journals. *Image: The Journal of Nursing Scholarship, 14,* 50–56.

Swanson, E., & McCloskey, J. C. (1982). The manuscript review process of nursing journals. *Image: The Journal of Nursing Scholarship, 14,* 72–76.

Chapter 12

Planning the Article

Deciding on Your Audience

Differences in format, emphasis, and tone mean that you must think carefully about which journal to send your article to (and remember, you can submit an article to only one journal at a time). Many people will advise you to decide on a journal before you begin and to write specifically for that journal. My advice is a little different. I think it is helpful, before you begin writing, to look at a few articles in the journals that you like and in which your article might be appropriate, to get a general notion of what your article should look like. (Do not, however, look at articles on your particular subject; that's too intimidating.)

When you come upon articles that impress you, look closely at the format and examine the contents. How long is the introduction? What points does it make? Is the purpose of the study given in the opening sentence or the closing sentence of the introduction? Is there a separate section on the theoretical framework? How detailed are the methods? How much is said about the analyses? How many tables are included? How is the closing discussion organized? How long is it? Is the tone formal or informal?

This information can help you see how to shape your own article and tell you what journals it will fit into. That's good to know at the outset. But it can be constricting to write with a particular journal before you; what is really important is not a definite format or style but a sense of your audience. That audience may spread over several journals, and you don't want to limit yourself to just one of them. For example, depending on its tone and focus, an article reporting a study of medication-taking among the elderly seen in a rural health clinic might be publishable in a nursing research journal, any one of several journals focusing on geriatric nursing or gerontology, a public health journal, or a general interest journal.

To decide who your audience is, ask yourself for whom your study might be important. Who needs to know what you have to report? Who can make best use of your findings? Sometimes you know very well that a study is likely to interest only one group of people—say, operating room nurses. But depending on how you conducted the study and what you found, that same study might also interest other nurse researchers, or people who educate operating room nurses, or administrators in the hospitals where those operating room nurses work. The audience for your article depends in part on the message you want to convey, the thrust of your article.

The Thrust of the Article

Research reports tend to be flat. They have no peaks and valleys, no moments of exciting discovery. That is because usually they have no focus. Completeness and clarity are their virtues, not sharpness of illumination. Articles, in contrast, cannot cover everything; no journal has the space to print everything that comes out of a study, and no reader has the patience to wade through it all. So when you begin an article you must choose what to emphasize, what to play down, and what to leave out altogether. In other words, you must decide on the thrust of the article: the most important thing you have to communicate.

If you set out with definite expectations and found what you were looking for, your findings are probably the most important information you have; everything in the article should point logically towards them, and you should give them greatest coverage. Suppose, however, that you found the opposite of what you expected; probably you'll still want to emphasize your findings, but you will need to give even more space to discussing why you found them.

Perhaps what matters most about your study is not the findings but a method you developed for measuring something: job satisfaction of nurses or the intensity of the pain patients experience after major surgery. That's what is important to explain in detail; your findings are important only because they provide the evidence for whatever you are discussing. At the other extreme, your findings may show that a generally respected method of measuring something is not so discriminating as had been thought. In that case, the emphasis will be on how you used the measurement tool, for the reader will want to know whether yours was a valid test of its merit. Or perhaps what is important is the ease with which other nurses can do what you did to improve the spirits of patients with end-stage renal disease; if so, you need to concentrate on explanations of how to put the treatment into practice.

As these examples illustrate, there are many ways to focus a research article. The focus or thrust you select will in part determine the audience for the article, just as the audience in part determines the thrust. What you and the audience consider important are the two markers that help you see where the article ought to go, that give it a unity of purpose. You may know those right away, and even the particular journal for which your article is best suited. In that case, query the journal as to interest (see Part Four, pages 200–202, for suggestions on writing a query), and request a copy of its guidelines for authors before you begin writing the article. Whenever those guidelines differ from the suggestions given here, follow the journal's rules.

Often, however, what you have to say and to whom you want to say it aren't clear at once. At first you see "through a glass darkly"; then slowly, in the act of describing what you dimly see, you find that the image grows plainer. As you begin to make the meaning clear, this clarity pushes your thinking further and you discover what it is you have to communicate. That is part of the excitement of writing: as you write, you think. That is also why it is hard to write a good research article (or any other kind of article) in one draft. You need to be able to go back and in a second draft make sure that all the parts fit together and everything is consistent with the thrust. Otherwise, the first half of the article may go one way and the second another because you figured out the essence of what you had to say when you were already halfway through the writing. And finally, that is why in many cases it's best to draft an article before deciding on which journal to submit it. Writing to someone else's specifications can constrict your thinking. Once your thrust is clear, it is not difficult to adapt your format and tone to fit the requirements of most journals.

Which Article to Write First?

Research articles are short, usually 10 to 15 double-spaced typed pages, almost never more than 18 or 20 pages, including references. But theses, dissertations, and research reports are long and often contain enough material for two or three articles that might be written for different audiences with different emphases. Before you begin to write, decide whether you have one article or two that you might write for different journals.

If you can write more than one, it's usually best to begin with the article that is closest to a standard report of your research, the one that describes methods with some completeness and summarizes major findings. Until you write that article, it will get in the way of any other article you want to write. You'll find yourself saying more than you want to about methods or findings that are not relevant to your thrust, simply because the information is there waiting to be communicated. Once the standard article is done, the problem disappears. You can leave unsaid what does not suit your purpose and simply refer readers to the article you've already written, thus: "The study methods are described more fully in Jane Doe, 'An Investigation of Nurses' Attitudes Toward Potential Drug Addiction in Patients.'"

If you write two or more articles from the same study, you must be careful not to repeat the same information over and over in different publications. Minor overlaps and repetitions are permissible, but generally the data should differ, not just the emphasis and tone. Unfortunately, it is not uncommon to find the same data presented again and again; in the long run that kind of publishing will advance neither nursing knowledge nor your career. So resist the temptation to repeat yourself.

The Literature Review

When you decide on the thrust of the article, you are almost ready to begin writing. But first you must go back to the library to see what has been published since you last looked. If you are writing from a thesis, dissertation, or research report that you have just completed, probably you don't have to worry. But if you finished the research longer ago than yesterday or did not make an extensive literature review before beginning, it's worth taking a new look at the literature. If what you have to say has now been said by someone else, there's no point in wasting your time. But because so much research done by nurses lies unpublished in dark desk drawers, there's a good chance that little new has been said since you completed your investigation. You are still the latest authority.

Even if more has been published, it's quite likely to differ substantially from what you have to say and thus leave ample room for your discussion of the subject. Even in the rare case when another researcher has published a study whose findings are close to your own, you often can refocus your article, direct it toward a different audience, and still publish.

You will, of course, need to take into account the new publications, either in your introduction or in the discussion of your own findings. The new information may actually strengthen your case. Don't be concerned if other researchers disagree with you; if, when you reexamine your study, you are convinced you have something to say, it's probably worth publishing. But it would be wise to say it soon, for there may be others preparing to say it, also.

And while you're saying it, don't look back at the literature again; it's too intimidating. Wait until you've finished a first draft of the article; then check once more if you feel you need to.

Chapter 13

The Standard Research Article

This chapter describes the content of a fairly standard research article. Such an article follows the organization of a thesis or dissertation, though it's much shorter. The article might appear in any number of journals, as you'll see from the quoted examples. When they're helpful, use those examples as models, but don't be constricted by them. The intent here is to provide guidelines, not rigid rules for writing. When the logic of your study conflicts with the guidelines, trust your own interpretations. (The next chapter deals with converting your original report into an article and so partially duplicates the content of this one, which is longer and more specific. Choose the chapter that better suits your purpose.)

Introduction and Literature Review

The first section of an article is brief, often only a few paragraphs. Its function is to provide a rationale and context for the study. This introductory section begins with a description of the problem, then quickly reviews the literature reporting work already done on the problem, notes gaps in that work, and concludes with a statement of purpose or an overview of the study.

Here is a succinct introduction to an article (McLendon, Fulk, & Starnes, 1982, p. 7) published in *JOGN Nursing*. It quickly establishes the problem and the need for the study being reported, then concludes with the purpose:

> Since cancer of the breast is the most common neoplasm and leading cause of cancer death in women, it is crucial to combat the disease by diagnosing it in an early stage through breast self-examination (BSE) and regular check-ups. Although BSE is a simple, painless, cost-free procedure requiring only a few minutes per month, studies have shown that the majority of American women fail to practice it with any regularity.[1-5] However, Mahoney found that after teaching the examination in a hospital breast clinic, 90% of the patients were performing the examination with competence and confidence.[6] Thus, Mahoney suggests that BSE, when done correctly, may be as useful as an annual breast examination performed by a physician.
>
> In a survey of 122 middle-class, predominantly Jewish women, Stillman found that although almost all were knowledgeable about BSE and believed it to be beneficial in improving early detection of breast cancer, few actually practiced BSE regularly, and many expressed doubt about their ability to perform the technique correctly. To encourage practice of self-examination, Stillman suggested that BSE be taught on a one-to-one basis by a nurse or physician, allowing time for questions and a demonstration of technique by the patient. The effectiveness of his strategy, however, had not been studied systematically.
>
> The purpose of this study was to assess the effect of one-to-one BSE teaching on retention of knowledge and accuracy of performance. Since members of low socioeconomic classes most often fail to engage in preventive health practices, such as breast self-examination, the teaching was implemented with this population.[7-10]

A review of the literature helps to establish the rationale for the study; logically, therefore, it should be incorporated into the introductory section, not separated from problem and purpose. Some journals, however, do handle it separately following the introduction. However you handle it, keep it short. Journals are always pressed for space. They sometimes publish review articles that summarize recent research on a topic, discuss the unresolved issues, and offer directions for further study. Except for review articles, editors and readers want just enough information about others' work to provide a context for your study and to show that it was needed—in short, to make it seem worth reading about.

In the article quoted above, for example, the authors refer generally to studies that show the majority of American women fail to practice breast self-examination regularly; this helps to establish the problem. Then they discuss a study showing that with proper teaching women could perform the examination competently and confidently, and they note that one author has suggested a teaching strategy that should be effective. They conclude by pointing out that the effectiveness of this strategy has not been studied systematically and thus they pave the way for their own study, whose purpose was to provide just such a systematic study.

To provide a context, the review of the literature should present the findings of the studies most closely related to your own. And, to show that your study was needed, it should point out the shortcomings of those other studies that limit the credibility or generalizability of their findings.

If there are no studies directly related to your own, as is often the case, the review must show your logic in building on other, apparently peripheral work. It should clearly point to gaps in the research. Here's a nice example of a review from *Geriatric Nursing* (Bassett, McClamrock, & Schmelzer, 1982, p. 103) that brings together work on the effects of exercise on flexibility, balance, and strength in various muscle groups to develop an argument for studying the effects of exercise on shoulder, hip, and knee flexibility; balance; and quadriceps strength in the elderly.

> Some older adults have decreased muscle strength, diminished endurance, and difficulty in restoring balance. These changes are thought to be the result of deconditioning and therefore amenable to improvement by exercise. Little research has been done, however, on the specific relationship of exercise to balance or to the musculoskeletal system in elderly people.
>
> Various researchers have examined the effects of exercise on flexibility of the ankle and hamstring (1), spine (1,2), index finger (3), and trunk (4,5). However, we found only one study, by Lesser, of shoulder, hip, and knee flexibility, all equally necessary for walking and ADL (6).
>
> Lesser showed that exercise improved shoulder flexion, which is necessary to reach items on a shelf, hang up clothes, and dress. She found no improvement in hip flexion and questionable improvement in knee flexion; both are involved in getting in and out of a chair or bathtub.

Of the three studies reviewed on the effects of exercise on balance in elders, none showed any change (4,5,7). The results of exercise to strengthen the quadriceps muscle, used in walking and getting in and out of a chair or bathtub, apparently have not been studied, but strength in other muscle groups has been shown to improve slightly with exercise (3,8,9).

Notice how the first paragraph establishes the specific problem and the lack of research on it, and the next three paragraphs review related research. First the authors discuss flexibility in areas that they are not interested in, then they focus on the one study of shoulder, hip, and knee flexibility. Next they mention three studies of balance that showed no change. Finally, they point out that nothing has been done on quadriceps strength though other muscles have improved with exercise. The discussion clearly establishes the need for a study of the effect of exercise on the variables they consider important for walking and other activities of daily living.

Many studies have no clear relation to theory. Even when they do the theoretical framework may not need to be articulated. For example, if your study and those that preceded it investigated the effects of a nursing intervention on patients' ability to handle the stress of illness or treatment, it is not necessary to review Selye's stress theory to establish the context for the studies. The introductory section might include a reference to Selye, but you can assume that readers understand his theory. Articles differ in this respect from theses and dissertations, in which you present the theoretical underpinnings for your argument not to inform your readers but to assure them that *you* are informed. Journal readers will assume that you know your bases, just as you assume they do.

When the theory your work is based on is new or little known or poorly understood, however, it is wise to explain it to readers. You also need to explain the theoretical basis for your work if the logic of your intervention or hypotheses would not otherwise be clear.

Here, for example, are excerpts from a discussion (Pierce & Thompson, 1976, pp. 14–15) of the theory behind a strategy for changing nursing practice, working through the department of inservice education. Without this discussion readers would have had no idea why the particular strategy was used. The article was published in the *Journal of Nursing Administration*.

Planned change has several interacting components: the environment in which it is to occur, the actual procedural technological variation from the existing to the desired practice, the human element that needs to be modified (the change target), the change agent, and the means for promoting and maintaining the revision.

In assessing the change environment, Kurt Lewin conceptualizes the "present state" as a dynamic equilibrium of driving and restraining forces (1). The forces are of two types, those that stem from the organizational/structural nature of the environment and those that accrue from the individual/personal interplay with the environment. To revise the present state, the dynamic equilibrium between the driving and restraining elements must be moved. . . .

Even if the proposed modification is of a procedural/technological nature, it is as important to consider social/organization and individual factors as when the focus is on altering human behavior (2). Sequential models have been developed for planned change that provide a framework for working with structural and individual behaviors in promoting a procedural change (3,4,5). . . .

Two models emphasize the interpersonal aspects of change by stressing the need for collaborative goalsetting (6,7). Schein points out, however, that there is difficulty in establishing and maintaining this collaborative relationship since most improvements require divergence from firmly established behaviors (8). Revising these behaviors tends to be emotionally resisted because the notion of change implies inadequacy of previous behaviors and/or practices, a conclusion which the change-target would naturally be motivated to reject. Approaches to overcoming this inherent resistance center on seeking and maintaining the active involvement of the change-target in the proposed modification while guaranteeing that there will be no resulting loss in his autonomy (9).

In the first paragraph the authors posit that planned change has four components; in subsequent paragraphs they review the theoretical bases for dealing with each of these components. Then, in the next section of the article (not shown here) they outline a strategy for improving nursing care based on this theoretical framework.

The theoretical framework is not usually presented under a separate heading. Theoretical work, like empirical work, is part of the literature and the two are reviewed together. If your conceptualization is clear, readers will recognize your study's relation to the theories presented without needing to be cued in by a heading.

The theoretical framework should come before the discussion of empirical studies if it also served as the basis for these studies.

If other authors approached the problem from a different perspective, however, describe their work before presenting the theoretical basis for your own study.

The introductory section concludes with a sentence or two giving the purpose of the study or an overview of the study methods. Here is a good example of a purpose statement concluding the introduction to an article published in *Cancer Nursing* (Wagner & Bye, 1979, p. 366).

> Alopecia represents a threat to body image and thus might be expected to arouse anxiety and result in restriction of social activities.[9] This study was designed to determine how alopecia affects the body image and social activity level of individuals receiving cancer chemotherapy.

Methods

Overview and Hypotheses or Research Questions.   The "Methods" section of an article must give readers who know nothing about the study enough information to convince them of the credibility of the findings and no more. The section usually begins with a one- or two-sentence overview of the study methods. This quick summary tells readers what was done to whom in order to find out what, and it serves as a framework for details to come. The following is a good overview found in *Heart & Lung* (Hoffman, Donckers, & Hauser, 1978, p. 804):

> This study was designed to assist nurses to intervene with and reduce stress perceived by patients in a CCU. The investigators questioned CCU patients about stress after their discharge from the unit and, on the basis of this information, conducted an in-service class that emphasized those stressors thought to be directly alterable by nursing intervention. The effectiveness of the program was evaluated by comparing the amount of stress perceived by patients before and after the in-service class.

In this article the introductory section does not conclude with a purpose statement. Instead the authors begin the overview by stating the purpose of their work; then they say what they did to whom and how they evaluated its effectiveness. Readers are thus prepared for what's to come.

An article does not include a schematic representation of the research design, and usually it is not even necessary to identify the type of design; one assumes that readers can do that themselves from the information given in the overview.

The overview may or may not be followed by hypotheses or research questions, depending on the formality of the article. If hypotheses are included, they are introduced in the past tense and written in the present or future tense; or they can be written in a combination of the past and conditional tenses. Here are examples of two styles (Grandjean, Bonjean, & Aiken, 1982, p. 30; Robarge, Reynolds, & Groothius, 1982, p. 200), both from *Research in Nursing and Health*.

> In the present research, the following hypotheses were examined: (a) centralization of decision-making is associated negatively with overall satisfaction; (b) the effect of centralization is most negative for faculty members with the strongest desires for autonomy.

> The following retrospective study was designed to test the hypothesis that a higher potential for abuse might exist following the birth of twins.

Hypotheses can also be presented less formally, as expectations. Here's an example from the study of alopecia quoted earlier:

> It was expected that subjects with alopecia would have a more negative body image and show a greater decrease in social activities than those without alopecia (Wagner & Bye, 1979, p. 366).

However they are written, hypotheses must always point to an expected association between variables, as in the study of centralized decision-making; or they must point to an expected difference between groups, as in the alopecia study and the study of child abuse in families with twins. Hypotheses are never written in the null form in an article and come immediately after the overview.

Like hypotheses, research questions are introduced in the past tense, then stated in the present or future tense. This excerpt from

Advances in Nursing Science illustrates (O'Connell et al., 1984, p. 22):

> Two specific questions were addressed in the study:
> 1. Do type II diabetic patients use symptoms to distinguish high, low, and normal blood glucose levels?
> 2. Do type II diabetic patients take action on symptoms as the model predicts?

Research questions are formal, like hypotheses. To make a presentation less formal, the questions can be omitted and the ideas conveyed indirectly through the overview or purpose statement. If research questions are included, they come immediately after the overview.

Occasionally an article has both hypotheses and research questions, but they are never on precisely the same topic. You would not, for example, first ask whether cancer patients with alopecia have a more negative body image than patients who have not lost their hair and then turn around and hypothesize that they do. That wastes words. If your study had hypotheses and also asked some additional, exploratory questions about matters you knew too little to hypothesize about, first present the hypotheses, then the additional questions.

Setting and Sample.   In an article the type of setting is identified, but its characteristics are described only to the extent that they will be important in helping readers understand or evaluate the sample obtained there and the findings about that sample. Use a name only if it adds relevant information, and then only with permission.

What follows is a brief, clear description of the setting in *The American Journal of Maternal Child Nursing* (Jackson, Bradham, & Burwell, 1978, p. 104):

> The study was conducted on a 10-bed ward completely composed of private rooms with individual bathrooms and beds for parents. This setting provided uniform opportunities for parents to participate in child care.

Notice how the authors describe only those aspects of the setting that point to opportunities for parental care (private rooms, pri-

vate baths, beds for parents), carefully noting that those opportunities were uniform. Any other information about the setting
would be irrelevant for this study.

If two or more settings were used, give parallel information
about them all. In other words, if you describe the type of rooms on
one unit, describe them on the other units so that readers can see
whether and to what extent the settings were equivalent.

The sample is described after the setting. The description
should include (1) the method of sample selection, (2) criteria for
selection, and (3) the method of assigning subjects to groups if
there were groups. The procedures followed in approaching subjects and gaining their consent to participate are often also described here, instead of being held back for a separate section
titled "Procedures," but details are omitted.

The sample section may include information on the potential
or initial sample size and the final number included in the analysis,
with explanations for any difference. The following description
(Knaje, 1982, p. 14), from *Research in Nursing and Health*, includes
the procedures and information on sample size along with criteria
for selection. The statement "Eighty-one sets of parents who met
these criteria were approached . . ." also makes clear the method of
selection.

> To participate in the study, parents had to have a child who was
> between 5 and 12 years old, expected to recover completely, expected
> to be hospitalized for no more than 10 days, and suffering from no
> major impairments other than the one for which the child was hospi-
> talized. Eighty-one sets of parents who met these criteria were ap-
> proached and asked to participate; seventy couples signed consent
> forms indicating their willingness to participate. Five couples subse-
> quently withdrew from the study. Of the remaining 65 couples, six
> were experiencing the hospitalization of an only child, so sibling
> response was not an issue. This report is based on data from the
> remaining 59 sets of parents.

Sometimes the sample characteristics are also described here.
This excerpt (Scott, 1983, p. 25) from *Nursing Research* combines
criteria and other characteristics to give all the information on the
sample at the beginning of "Methods"

> Eighty-five women admitted to a large, urban cancer center for sur-
> gical biopsy to ascertain presence of carcinoma of the breast were

included in the study. Subjects were between the ages of 18 and 60, with educational levels ranging from high school through college; socioeconomic levels ranged from 1 through 6 according to the Hamburger classification (1957). Subjects voluntarily consented to take part in the study and were able to participate in and tolerate the testing of cancer and all were afebrile on both testing occasions.

Intervention. If the study included an intervention, it should be described clearly enough so that readers can judge whether it was adequate to bring about the desired effect. In most cases it isn't necessary to give a lot of detail; nursing interventions are rarely so precise or controlled as to require exact replication. The aim in an article is to allow readers to evaluate the treatment and adapt it for their own settings, not to enable them to duplicate the work. The more controlled the intervention and the more precisely defined the difference between groups, the more complex the evaluation, and the more exact must be any replication, and, therefore, the more details you need to give.

Below are two very different descriptions of interventions, both quite appropriate. The first, from *Pediatric Nursing* (Adams, 1982, p. 29), is brief and general:

> Using lecture format with a slide presentation, the investigator presented two classes to the experimental group on the importance of wearing seat belts, the way they work, the correct way to put on and take off a seat belt, and the safest way for a child to ride in the car. In addition, a homework assignment was given between the sessions.

The second description, from *Nursing Research* (Brooten et al., 1983, p. 226), is complex and detailed (only excerpts are given here):

> Group I received bromocriptine mesylate 2.5 mg twice a day for 14 days. In addition, they received, as did Groups II, III, and IV, the hospital's standard instructions for nonbreastfeeding postpartum mothers. These included wearing their own brassiere (except women in Group II for the duration of the hospital stay), avoiding stimulation to their breasts, applying ice as needed for discomfort and requesting analgesics as needed for breast pain.
> Group II wore a standard tight-fitting bra (nylon and cotton, Mary Jane Co., style #481). The bra, applied in the recovery room immediately postdelivery, completely covered the breast area, had adjustable straps, and two rows of four clips in the back....
> Group III had fluids limited to body-maintenance requirements

using the formula of Brooks (1968) (1500 ml/M²/day). Each woman recorded her fluid intake for seven days. To assist with this process, she was given two plastic drinking cups, a 12-ounce cup for hot fluids and a 14-ounce cup for cold fluids.

Group IV had a standardized compression binder applied in the recovery room. The binder was a uniform postsurgical abdominal support, ten inches wide (Scott Specialties, style #5738-2844).

The description of the intervention is often followed by a sentence indicating how its effectiveness was assessed. For example, in the study of seat belt usage quoted earlier, the description of the educational program concludes thus:

> Effectiveness was measured by comparing the knowledge of belt usage and the reported use of seat belts by the 48 children who received the educational program with that reported by 62 children in the control group who did not receive the program (Adams, 1982, p. 29).

Sometimes the procedure for taking subjects through the intervention and through pre- and/or posttesting is also described here, instead of in a later, separate section headed "Procedure."

Data Collection.   If the study included an intervention, the section on the measurement of variables tells how the intervention was evaluated. If the study had no intervention, this section tells what data were collected and how, in order to test the study hypotheses or answer the research questions.

The section begins with an introductory sentence or two indicating what variables were measured or what tools were used to collect what types of data. Then each tool is described separately. The section generally describes the most important or most precise measurements first and then moves to the less important or more general tools. Thus, physiological measurements come first, then scheduled observations, and finally questionnaires or interviews. When there are two or more tools of the same type—two questionnaires, say—the one that gave the most precise or important information is described first, then the others, always moving toward the more general.

The tools should be introduced in the order in which they are described so that readers are prepared for what's ahead. A good introduction to the data collection section comes from *Cancer Nursing* (Wall & Gabriel, 1983, p. 448):

> Four tools were used to collect information about the children's taste: materials for testing taste acuity, a questionnaire to assess changes in food preferences in children with leukemia, a questionnaire to document food preferences in healthy children, and an interview schedule for all children concerning food likes and dislikes.

Note that a physiological measure is mentioned first, then a questionnaire on the subjects of particular interest: children with leukemia, next a questionnaire on the comparison group, and finally a more general interview schedule for both groups. The tools are described in the same order.

If the sample characteristics beyond those constituting criteria for inclusion in the study are described in the "Setting and Sample" section, collection of these data is not mentioned here, for it's after the fact. Often, however, sample characteristics that might affect the variables of interest are described at the beginning of "Findings" or in connection with the particular findings they might affect. In such cases collection of these data is described at the end of the section on tools (though this need not be mentioned in the introduction). For example, in the article on taste changes just quoted, the section on tools concludes thus (Wall & Gabriel, 1983, p. 449):

> The following information was obtained from the leukemic children's charts: drug protocol, type of leukemia, date of diagnosis, number of relapses, status at time of testing (remission or relapse), and any other medical problems of the child.

The description of a tool must enable readers to evaluate its adequacy in obtaining the desired information. If it's a new tool or one that's little known, obviously it needs to be described in some detail. For physiological measurements, tell the data sought, the instrument used, and the time and manner of use and recording. For scheduled observations, tell precisely what was observed and when; if precision was impossible, give the criteria used to interpret what you saw. (If others made the observations, tell how you trained them and assured yourself that they were consistent in their interpretations.) Here's an example from the *AANNT Journal* of the kind of information needed to show how observations are interpreted (Lowrey & Femea, 1984, p. 28):

> Dialyzer clotting was determined both objectively and subjectively. Subjectively, if the dialyzer appeared to be clotted after the treatment was terminated, clotting was said to have occurred. Objectively, clotting was said to have occurred if any of the following conditions were met:
>
> 1. The dialyzer arterial pressure increased 50mmHg or more and the venous pressure decreased 50mmHg or more.
> 2. The post-transfusion ACT level was less than 150.
> 3. The post-transfusion ACT level was less than one and a half times the baseline level.

For questionnaires or interviews, first tell the topics covered and the types of questions; you may also need to include a couple of sample questions for greater clarity. Here's a good description of a questionnaire given to terminally ill patients and their families from an article in the *American Journal of Nursing* (Putnam et al., 1980, pp. 1451–1452):

> The questionnaires for patients and family members were similar. Patients were asked:
>
> where they wanted to be cared for during the terminal stages of their diseases and where they wanted to die;
>
> the major factors influencing their preference;
>
> possible influencing factors chosen from a list compiled by the investigators and the most important factor from this list;
>
> what services they thought would be needed if they preferred to die at home;
>
> the most important service from a list of possible services compiled by the investigators.
>
> Finally, a hypothetical situation describing support systems that could be made available (for example, a professional nurse, who could be called at any hour, public health nurses to help with physical care, and access to needed equipment and medications) was presented, and patients were asked if the availability of these services would influence their choice of place of death.

Note that the authors indicate all the major types of information sought but do not give details or examples except in one instance where readers might not otherwise know what they're talking about (in the discussion of "support systems").

If an instrument is widely known, it is not necessary to describe it. For example, look at this description from *Research in Nursing and Health* (Jordan & Meckler, 1982, p. 74):

> The Anderson College Schedule of Recent Experience (CSRE), which was used to measure life change events in this study, is similar to the life change instruments developed by Holmes and Rahe (Rahe, 1978), but was tailored to college students (Marx, Garrity, & Bowers, 1975). To fit the present sample, minor modifications were made on three items. Students were asked to indicate the number of times each event occurred during the past 6 months and then to determine a subjective life change unit value (LCU) on a scale of 0 to 100 to indicate the amount of personal adaptation demanded for that event (Rahe, 1978). A subjective life change score was obtained for each subject by multiplying the number of occurrences of each event by the subjective LCU and summing the results.

Note that the instrument is not described at all; the authors merely indicate that it is similar to other life change instruments and point out that minor modifications were made for their sample. Then they move on to how the instrument was used and scored.

After a note about use and scoring, the description of a questionnaire or scale concludes with a statement about whether validity and reliability have been established. If it's another's tool, there is usually no need to tell *how* these were established. You need to give details only if later you will discuss problems you encountered with the tool. This is a good example of what's needed from *AORN Journal* (Kathol, 1984, p. 134):

> The Spielberger State Anxiety Inventory was used to measure family member anxiety. This inventory consists of 20 statements that allow the respondents to rate their present feelings of anxiousness on a scale ranging from one to four, with one indicating no anxiousness and four indicating high anxiety. Spielberger et al. established construct validity, concurrent validity, and test-retest reliability for this inventory.[13]

Note that the last statement is referenced so that readers who want the information on how validity and reliability were established can get it.

If you developed a questionnaire yourself, describe any pilot tests or other efforts you made to establish validity and reliability of the tool, since these will affect the credence readers give to your findings. Be brief but give reasonably complete information.

Procedure. If the procedures used to acquire subjects and take them through the intervention and testing are particularly complex, they may be described in a separate section at the end of "Methods." Often, however, the research procedures are incorporated into other sections describing the study methods, with no separate section headed "Procedure." For example, a previously quoted article integrates tests and procedures in one chronological account of how subjects were identified and approached, gave consent to participate, had blood drawn, and were interviewed:

> Subjects identified by a prescreening chart review were contacted by telephone the afternoon or evening prior to the clinic appointment by either the secretary or one of the investigators; a telephone script was used to decrease variability in subject information and expectations. Subjects were contacted in person the following morning to give informed consent, to have venous blood drawn for subsequent C-peptide determination, and to participate in a structured interview lasting 30 to 60 minutes.
>
> The interview consisted of questions about former and current diabetes treatment methods and their duration; methods of determining glucose levels at home; use of symptoms in determining high, low, and normal glucose levels; specific symptoms used; confidence in the accuracy of these symptoms; action taken on the symptoms; and perception of whether action taken was effective (O'Connell et al., 1984, p. 23).

Definitions. In an article there's no need for a section called "Definitions" or "Definition of Terms." You can assume that readers understand all the terms you will use except any that are new or used in a special way. Any terms that need defining should be defined in context the first time they are used, whether that is in the literature review or in the section on methods or findings. What follows is a good illustration of the way to give definitions:

> Taste acuity was measured using the Henkin method of determining detection and recognition thresholds for each taste quality. Detection threshold is the lowest concentration of a given solution that a person

recognizes as different from distilled water; recognition threshold is the concentration at which a person can correctly identify the taste of the solution (Wall & Gabriel, 1983, p. 448).

Findings

The study findings are organized like this: first the sample is described if that was not done earlier; then the data are presented; next come tests of significance, if applicable; and finally exploratory or further analyses. Depending on the complexity of the methods and findings, an introductory sentence may be needed to remind readers of the major information sought, as in this article from the *Journal of Nursing Education* (Friesen & Stotts, 1984, p. 186):

> This study examined the effect of two teaching methods on the retention of CPR cognitive knowledge and psychomotor skills of baccalaureate nursing students. Mean scores for retention of cognitive knowledge in BCLS (basic cardiac life support) were compared; there was no difference in retention between the two methods.

Note that this article does not give sample characteristics here but moves straight from the introductory sentence to the major findings.

Description of the Sample.   The sample is frequently described at the beginning of "Findings," but only information that will be useful for evaluating the findings should be included. Begin by giving the potential and actual sample sizes, with explanations for the difference between them, and then describe any sample characteristics that might affect the findings or will be interesting in themselves. If study groups differed significantly in any of these characteristics, say so here to prepare readers for possible effects (nonsignificant differences should not be mentioned unless they seem to you practically important). Here's a concise sample from the *Western Journal of Nursing Research* (Osguthorpe, Roper, & Saunders, 1983, p. 210):

Two hundred and two men completed this study. Patients ranged in age from 20 to 64, with a mean of 39. The modal educational level was at the eighth to twelfth grade level (61%); the next highest education level was "some college" (29%); eighth grade and below (5%) and not stated (5%) were last. The ethnic–racial composition of the sample was as follows: 53.5% white, 40.1% black, 5.9% Hispanic-American and 0.5% other. Diagnostically, the majority of patients were categorized as psychotic (51%) with a minority of patients identified as mixed (20%), other (16%) or uncodable (13%). Neither age nor educational level was distributed evenly across the four groups. Groups C and D demonstrated an educational level that was significantly higher than the other two groups.

Description of the Data.   Always describe the study findings before discussing tests of the hypotheses or other statistical analyses. Tell what your measurements or observations showed, how subjects scored on tests, and what their responses were to questionnaires. This will prepare readers for tests of significance and for a discussion of what it all means.

If the study included an intervention, first give the important findings from the pretest or pre-intervention observations or measurements. If there was a comparison group, tell whether and how the experimental and comparison groups differed on these pre-intervention measures. Next give the corresponding post-intervention data and then point out the differences between pre- and post-figures. If there were groups, conclude by noting the differences in change in scores between the groups.

If the study did not include an intervention, give the most important and interesting findings first. If the most important findings were not central to the study purposes, first briefly present information on the variables the study focused on, then move quickly to the more interesting information.

Overall patterns, scores, or measurements always precede item analysis or detailed examination of the components of a measure. Here, for example, from *The Journal of Continuing Education in Nursing*, is the opening description of data from a survey of nurses to assess their perception of the importance of issues in professional nursing and health care delivery and to determine their interest in continuing education courses on a variety of topics (Philbrick, 1984, p. 206):

> All 26 professional nursing and health care delivery issues were rated as important or very important by at least 59% of the respondents,

and 19 of the 26 issues were deemed important or very important by at least 75% of the respondents. However, of the two groups of issues, the nursing issues were rated more important overall than were health care delivery issues. Six of the seven nursing issues were seen as important or very important by at least 85% of the respondents (Table 1). Of the broader health care issues, 13 were rated as important or very important by at least 75% of the respondents (Table 2).

The item rated important or very important by the most participants was "Nursing Education: Determining the knowledge and skills nurses need to meet the health care needs of patients" (Table 1).

Notice how the author first gives overall response patterns, then moves to particular issues. When mean scores are given, the range or standard deviation should be noted; readers may need to be reminded of the instrument's possible range as well.

Tables must be used sparingly in an article because they are expensive to typeset and consume a lot of space. Use them when you need to present a set of numbers that are crucial but would be so cumbersome in the narrative as to be unreadable; then simply give the major points in the text. Here's a description (Helton, Gordon, & Nunnery, 1980, p. 466) of findings with an accompanying table from *Heart & Lung*; note how the narrative highlights the main points while the table gives all the numbers.

The majority of the subjects (56%) were sleep deprived during the first day in the ICU. The percentage of the sample with sleep deprivation decreased with each subsequent day in the ICU; however, almost 20% of the subjects were still sleep deprived on the third day in the unit. In general, the pattern of sleep deprivation corresponded to the severity of the patient's condition. On day 1, 68% of the subjects were in unstable conditions, whereas by day 3 this percentage had declined to 26% (Table 1).

Table 1. Sleep deprivation, category of illness, and mental status of subjects for days 1 to 5 in ICU.

	Day in unit				
	1	2	3	4	5
No. of subjects	62	62	62	32	20
Mean sleep deprivation (%)	56	35	18	21	28
Mean cumulative sleep deprivation (%)	56	41	23	27	33
% sample in unstable condition	68	36	26	16	15
% sample with altered mental status	2*	5	11	9	10

*Subjected to ICU environment prior to entering study.

Hypothesis Testing.   If the data are complex and you have several hypotheses, hypothesis testing is best described after all the data are presented. The hypotheses should be woven into the narrative, and any maneuvers of the data needed to facilitate testing should be explained. Indicate the statistical procedure used to test for significance, but do not describe the procedure unless it is out of the ordinary or would normally be considered inappropriate for your data (in those cases you must explain what features of the test led you to select it). If included, the actual statistics are usually given in parentheses (and p is always italicized).

In a study with only one major hypothesis or perhaps a couple of closely related hypotheses, the most logical way to organize the findings is not to describe the data first and then discuss hypothesis testing but to combine hypothesis testing with the description. Begin by restating the hypothesis (i.e., the difference you expected to see between groups or the association between variables), unless that will be clear to readers from "Methods" or your introduction to "Findings." Next describe the data; give the raw scores or measurements or categorized responses or observations. Then tell whether there were any differences or associations and point out whether these were statistically significant. You can conclude by noting whether or not the data supported your hypothesis, or you can leave that conclusion to readers.

A good example of this organization is from the *Journal of Nurse Midwifery* (Yeates & Roberts, 1984, p. 7):

> It was hypothesized that the control group would report a more exhausting experience during the second stage of labor than the experimental group. Choice of responses on the interview questionnaire included exhausting, difficult, moderately difficult, came naturally, and effortless. No one responded that pushing was effortless and therefore this category was eliminated. A two-by-two contingency table was formed: category one consisted of exhausting and difficult; category two consisted of moderately difficult and came naturally. The Fisher's exact probability test was used to analyze the data. No difference was found between groups at the 0.05 level of significance.

Notice how the authors first give the hypothesis, weaving it smoothly into the narrative instead of plunking it down unceremoniously. Then they tell how they collapsed the data into two categories so they could test the hypothesis; next they name the statistical procedure they used; and finally they point out that they found no significant difference between groups. Clearly, the hypothesis was not supported.

When hypotheses were not supported and expectations thus not met, you can omit the hypotheses altogether, in both "Methods" and "Findings." Simply note that certain of the findings were unexpected and try to explain how and why they came about, as in this excerpt from *The Canadian Journal of Psychiatric Nursing* (Haber, Murphy, & Taylor, 1977, p. 9):

> There were no significant changes during the eight weeks for any of the groups in their levels of depression or activity (as measured by the SDS and KAS:FTA and KAS:SEA [Self-Rating Depression Scale, Katz Free Time Activity Scale and Katz Socially Expected Activity Scale]). Similarly, no significant changes were found on any of the additional psychological measures. Several explanations may account for these findings. The elderly may, due to hearing difficulties, require more time to begin functioning effectively as a group, so that an eight-week period was not long enough for resolution of depression within this population. Further, group members were not seeking treatment for identified problems; therefore, they may have been less motivated to gain something from psychotherapy. In any event, the information gained via self report tools was not valid because of the difficulties subjects had in completing the tools.

These authors give no hypotheses; they report the disappointing outcome of their intervention in two sentences, then offer three possible explanations for it.

Exploratory or additional, unplanned analyses of data conclude the findings section. Often the methods used and the reasoning behind these analyses need to be explained because the analyses, arising out of other findings, are not prepared for in "Methods."

Comments.   Whenever a finding is unexpected you should comment on it, as in the article on psychotherapy for the elderly just quoted; otherwise, readers will wonder if you understand the significance of what you found.

Comments also give depth to the findings and connect them to the real world. In the following excerpt from *Nursing Administration Quarterly* (Alt-White, Charns, & Strayer, 1983, p. 14), for example, the authors' comments turn an abstract term "communications process" into a description of the atmosphere on a unit:

> Three managerial factors also were found to be strongly related to nurse-physician collaboration. The first, communications process on the unit, reflects the degree to which communication on the unit is open, conflict is managed productively rather than avoided or smoothed over, and meetings are a useful forum for discussion. This finding is consistent with expectations that effective communication on a unit contributes to collaboration. The converse may also be true. When people are able to collaborate, the inherent trust in that working relationship contributes to the open and effective communication process.

Note how the authors are careful to point out that while the correlation they found fits with the idea that open communication contributes to collaboration, the cause-effect relationship may be going the other way.

Generally you should discuss the overall meanings of your findings in the concluding section of an article, but comment on particular findings as you go. That's because when you report a finding and save your comment for later, you have to repeat the finding to introduce the comment, and that can waste space and readers' time. Sometimes, however, it's impossible to divide comments neatly into two categories, particular and general. For example, the article quoted above is titled "Personal, Organizational and Managerial Factors Related to Nurse-Physician Collaboration," and, as the title warns, the study produced not a series of individual findings but groups of findings on each of the types of factors examined. The authors solved the problem that was created by combining "Results" and "Discussion" and commenting on individual findings as they fitted into the groups. Depending on the number and complexity of your findings, you may need to do that too.

Sometimes people hold their comments for the "Discussion" section, especially when little or no repetition is required to remind readers of the findings involved. Here's a case in point from *Oncology Nursing Forum* (Ingle, Burish, & Wallston, 1984, p. 100):

> A somewhat confusing finding was the high positive correlation between ANV [anticipatory nausea and vomiting] and coping effort,

indicating that the more conditioned a subject was, the more ways that subject tried to cope with having cancer. This conflicts with findings by Altmaier and others, who found that patients with ANV demonstrated significantly less desire and ability to cope.[5] One possible explanation is that conditioned subjects may have adopted an "I'll-try-anything-that-might-help" attitude, thus checking more coping statements, while those who were not conditioned may have had less need to try a large number of different coping strategies.

These comments are in the concluding section of the article; note how the authors quickly remind readers of the finding they are going to discuss, point out that it was confusing and in conflict with findings by other authors, and then speculate about possible explanations for the finding.

Whenever others have worked on a similar problem, you should comment on how your data fit with theirs. Indicate whether your findings are in conflict with others', as in the study above; whether they confirm others' findings; or whether and how they extend our understanding of what others have done. These comparisons can be made in commenting on particular findings or in the concluding discussion, wherever they seem most appropriate.

Anecdotal Data.   Like comments and explanations, anecdotal data give findings depth and relevance. They also provide support for numbers and add a human touch, a sense of the individuals who make up a numerical mean. In the following excerpt (Deberry, Jefferies, & Light, 1975, p. 2193) the authors use their observations of individuals to illustrate the range of improvement they found after teaching patients to manage their medications, and help explain that range:

> We observed that the patient's degree of motivation appeared particularly important. One patient, who did not have a first-grade education but who seemed eager to learn to take his own medicines, did extremely well on his post-test in comparison to his pre-test. Another patient, who had a Ph.D. degree, saw little purpose in learning about medicines and showed only slight improvement on his post-test.
>
>   The presence of family members during teaching sessions appeared to help motivate patients and reinforce our teaching. Often the family seemed as eager to learn as did the patient. One man's wife learned to note the dosage of her husband's prescription and to question discrepancies between the written instructions we had given them and the instructions received at the pharmacy.

In the first paragraph the importance of motivation is illustrated by a telling detail: the ignorant man improved more than the educated man. The second paragraph explains the role families played in motivation, using details about one man's wife to elaborate on that point. Such details make a description come alive and guarantee that readers will follow it. (Note that the article was published in the *American Journal of Nursing*; a more formal research journal would have been less likely to sanction the reference to the investigators in the first person ["we"].)

Anecdotal data can be reported wherever they seem most appropriate; if they add new information, however, it is best to include them in "Findings." The concluding discussion should not bring in new data, only new ideas.

Discussion

The Major Findings.   The final section of an article pulls everything together and shows what the study can mean to others. This concluding discussion should first summarize the major findings, but only the major ones; the aim is not to repeat the "Findings" section but to highlight study outcomes and make a claim for their importance. Here's a good example from *The Journal of Nursing Administration* (Vik & MacKay, 1982, p. 13):

> The results of this study suggest that the shift patterns worked by nurses do affect the care received by patients. Patients cared for by nurses who worked 8-hour shifts received better care, as measured by the QualPacs [Quality Patient Care Scale], than did patients cared for by nurses working 12-hour shifts.

Notice how the authors first make their claim—shift patterns do affect care—then they back this up with the major finding from their study.

Some authors go even further in stating the case for the importance of what they've found. Look at this passage from *Nursing Management* (Nelson, 1984, p. 39):

> The NHCU [Nursing Home Care Unit] experience and the year-long
> study which reviewed it demonstrated the value of some important
> notions about caring for chronically ill and disabled patients. A
> nursing coordinated, rehabilitation oriented, health team approach
> in a long-term care setting can prevent both extended hospitalization
> and undue institutionalization. In this system, the nurse manager, as
> coordinator, plays a key role in returning such patients to indepen-
> dent living. These findings confirm those of Kaplan et al., although in
> their study the social worker, rather than the nurse, coordinated the
> comprehensive health team approach.

This author generalizes the major findings immediately: the nurse-
coordinated team approach *can prevent* extended hospitalization;
the nurse coordinator *plays* a key role. Note also that the author
strengthens the claim for the findings by comparing them to those
of another investigator.

In the following from *Pediatric Nursing* (Aquilino & Ely, 1985,
p. 46), the authors make a more modest claim. First, they point out
that their findings contradict the general view that parents know
little about their children's sexual curiosity and activity and therefore react negatively to them. Then they note that in their sample
parents with more knowledge seemed to feel more comfortable,
but they are careful to say they found no significant correlations
between knowledge, responses, and comfort. Finally, they offer
one possible explanation: people said what they thought they
should say, rather than disclosing what they really did.

> While it is often believed that parents know little about the sexual
> curiosity and activity of 3 to 5 year olds and this lack of parental
> knowledge causes negative responses and discomfort, the majority of
> parents in this study were very knowledgeable and responded
> positively to situations involving normal preschool sexual activities.
> However, parental comfort with childhood sexuality varied. More
> knowledgeable parents reported greater comfort, yet there was no
> significant correlation between knowledge and response or between
> response and comfort. It is possible that parents in this study chose
> responses to items based on what they thought others would like for
> them to do, rather than disclosing what they would actually do.

Limitations.   The opening claim for the findings should be
followed by a discussion of limitations on their validity,
usefulness, or generalizability. (The discussion should be built
into the narrative, not set apart in a separate section titled "Limita-

tions.") When you mention a limitation, always say what it derives from and what it limits. It's also helpful to point out what would have been ideal methods and how you tried to get around the limitations of less than ideal methods. Conclude by saying why you don't think the limitations of the study are crippling, if that is the case.

Below is a good example from the study of shift patterns and their effect on patient care quoted a little earlier. In the first paragraph the authors point to two limitations on generalizability and then to a more serious limitation: the possible effects of uncontrolled variables on the variable they were measuring, quality of patient care. In the second paragraph, they describe a way of collecting the data—before and after the change in shift patterns— that would avoid the problem of these uncontrolled variables; then they explain why they couldn't do it that way and go on to describe the technique they used instead: matching units according to standard criteria. Note their conclusion: this technique was good enough to produce useful data.

> . . . we recognize some important limitations of the study. There was no control over specialized versus general units; and data were collected in only one hospital, thus limiting the generalization of results. Other variables which could not be controlled may have influenced patient care. They include the fact that patients took an early afternoon rest hour, the interaction of the head nurse with some patients, nurse fatigue, and the nurses' attitudes toward the 12-hour shift. In view of these limitations and influencing variables, we emphasize that the study findings must be interpreted with caution.
>
> Evaluation of the three 12-hour-shift units both before and after they switched to the 12-hour shift would have been ideal. At the time of the study, however, many of the units were on 12-hour shifts and the nursing administrative staff was averse to converting any more units before studying the effects of this shift pattern. The investigators felt that if the units were matched as closely as possible according to other established criteria, the results would be useful (Vik & MacKay, 1982, p. 13).

Suggestions for Further Research. The discussion of limitations leads naturally to suggestions for further research, since the studies proposed are usually aimed at overcoming the limitations of the present study (if it had no shortcomings, no limitations on its generalizability, there'd be no need for further research). Like limitations, these suggestions should be built into the discussion, not set apart in a special section.

Suggestions should be specific and concrete so that readers who might decide to do further studies can see clearly what needs to be done. The article on taste alterations in children with leukemia cited earlier provides a useful excerpt (Wall & Gabriel, 1983, p. 451).

> While taste changes were documented by this study along with some changes in food preferences, the complexity of the variables involved and the sometimes contradictory findings make it hard to explain fully the results. Longitudinal studies with larger sample sizes need to be done to assess more accurately the effects of the many variables that affect taste. A child's taste needs to be followed over the course of time, beginning at diagnosis and continuing as new drugs are added and deleted from the treatment regime. Growth and development charts along with height and weight changes would be necessary for complete assessment of nutritional status.

As is evident, these authors don't stop at suggesting longitudinal studies with larger samples; they also suggest looking at taste at the time of diagnosis and whenever drugs are changed, and looking at growth and development charts as well as weight and height changes. Suggestions like these will help another researcher design a study whose results can be more fully explained.

It's important to suggest doing *no* further research if your study indicates that further research will not be fruitful. Such suggestions can save other researchers valuable time and energy, which they can then invest in research with more potential. Here is such a suggestion from the study of the relationship between dysmenorrhea and life change events cited earlier (Jordan & Meckler, 1982, p. 78):

> In conclusion, while the correlations between life change and dysmenorrhea in this study were somewhat higher than those of Siegel et al. (1979), life change accounted for only a small percentage of the variance in MDQ [Menstrual Distress Questionnaire] scores (12%). Since in neither study was life change a good predictor of menstrual distress, the investigators feel that no further life change research involving dysmenorrhea is needed. In fact, the practicality of present life change tools must be questioned for any research problems, as the same pitfalls continue to be encountered. While recent revisions

of these instruments have expanded the number and type of events tapped, the predictive value of life change events for illness outcomes has not been demonstrated (Dohrenwend, Krasnoff, Ashkenasy, & Dohrenwend, 1978).

Life change events, say these authors, not only do not predict menstrual distress but, with present tools, do not predict any illness outcomes. Note, however, that while the authors recommend no further life change research involving dysmenorrhea, they stop short of saying there should be no further life change research at all, for that would go beyond the scope of their data; they could not support such a statement.

Implications for Theory.   If a study was not explicitly related to theory, there need be no mention of theory in the concluding section of the article. But if the study tested a theoretical proposition or was based on a theoretical model, this concluding discussion must make clear the study's implications for the theory; these points should come right after or together with the discussion of further research. Your findings may confirm the usefulness of the theory or model or raise questions about it. The data may also suggest a need for modifications in the theory, or they may indicate that it is not an accurate reflection of reality and needs to be discarded. Similarly, your study findings may show that the model you used needs some refining, or that it is not a useful conceptualization of the problem or solution. Don't shy away from such implications; they may be among the most important points you have to make.

The following discussion from *Nursing Research* (Toney, 1983, p. 19) points out the need for modifications in the theory of bonding, especially when applied to fathers:

> This study found no significant difference in bonding behaviors between fathers who had contact for ten minutes with their infants during the first hour following delivery and those who did not.
>
> The length of the sensitive period proposed by Klaus and associates (1972), the first few minutes and hours after birth, may be longer, including the first few days postpartum (Salk, 1970). In addition, the importance placed on a specific limited time for optimal bonding in all parents may be inflexible, neglecting each individual's ability for adaptation and the effects of variables surrounding new parents. Significance of the sensitive period may be more appropriately deter-

> mined for parents after evaluating their specific needs for bonding enhancement.
>
> Assuming that the sensitive period is similar in both parents may also be fallacious. . . .

Notice how the author first points out that no significant difference was found between fathers who held their babies right away and those who didn't. Then, on this basis, the author suggests that the theory of bonding may be too inflexible in its description of a "sensitive" period: the period may be longer than proposed, its significance may be less than proposed, and it may not be the same for mothers and fathers.

Implications for Practice.   The final paragraphs of an article should tell readers how the study findings can be used *now*— despite their limitations and despite any need for further research. These paragraphs draw conclusions from the data, point out the overall meanings of the study, and make practical suggestions for readers. Here's a good example from *Nurse Educator* (Schroeder, Cantor, & Kurth, 1981, pp. 16–17):

> The following are suggested by the data: (1) Educational programs have not identified the core content needed in the acute care setting. (2) Students tend to learn procedures rather than application of principles and concepts; the learning of such procedures is more a matter of clinical experience and teaching style than planned learning experiences. (3) Application of the nursing process for predicting and evaluating nursing care is poorly understood by new graduates.
>
> It seems clear that diagnostic testing would be the best way to plan the inservice educational programs for individuals. Needs are so varied it would be a waste to provide the same intructional content to all new employees. Also, it would be dangerous to withhold content from individuals on the basis of previous clinical experience. Carefully developed diagnostic tests, however, can determine the inservice program required by each new staff member.
>
> The success of such testing depends on two factors: the predictive ability of the tests and the flexibility of the inservice program. It will be necessary for individual students to participate in different instructional units. This approach, however, will not work if all students are locked into a predetermined curriculum. Also important is the ability of the inservice educators to select essential content and the most efficient method for presenting it.
>
> The following recommendations should help students develop the content base needed for correct patient care decisions: (1) Each

inservice educational program should develop a core of content relevant to decisions about patients, not content related to hospital routines and practices nor restricted to the acquisition of manipulative skills.

Look at how the authors move from their conclusion that there are three general types of deficits in the preparation of new graduates to the first step in their solution: diagnostic testing to determine the deficits of individuals. Then they offer the rest of the solution: a series of recommendations for overcoming these deficits through inservice programs.

Readers are looking for practical suggestions like these, ways to do better what they are doing, ways to improve education, administration, and practice—ultimately, ways to improve the care of patients.

Sometimes, however, the important suggestion is "do nothing." Examine the excerpt from *The Nurse Practitioner* (Ervin, Komaroff, Baranowski, & Pass, 1982, p. 21):

> Despite these limitations and the clear need for additional research, there seems little current reason to advise women to alter their hygienic, sexual, or clothing practices to prevent vaginal infection. In the individual woman with recurrent vaginitis which seems clearly related to a particular practice, specific advice about discontinuation of that practice might well be indicated.

Whatever your conclusions and recommendations, the final paragraph should be clear, convincing, and, if possible, catchy. Look at this paragraph from *Nursing & Health Care* (Smith, Jepson, & Perloff, 1982, p. 98):

> With hospital costs continuing to spiral upward, and with the number of elderly people increasing daily, there is no alternative to preparing all health care providers for elderly patients. Hence, selection and training of nursing care providers who *care* is one way to meet the needs effectively and efficiently. As Francis Peabody said, "The secret of the care of the patient is caring for the patient."

The authors make a strong statement about the need for providers who care. But it is the play on words in the last sentence that gives the extra punch. That's the kind of conclusion that satisfies readers; they go away from the article convinced of the point, and pleased with it, too. No author could ask for more.

References

Adams, D. (1982). Children's response to a belt restraint program. *Pediatric Nursing, 8,* 28-30.

Alt-White, A. C., Charns, M., & Strayer, R. (1983). Personal, organizational and managerial factors related to nurse-physician collaboration. *Nursing Administration Quarterly, 8,* 8-18.

Aquilino, M. L., & Ely, J. (1985). Parents and the sexuality of preschool children. *Pediatric Nursing, 11,* 41-46.

Bassett, C., McClamrock, E., & Schmelzer, M. (1982). A 10-week exercise program for senior citizens. *Geriatric Nursing, 3,* 103-105.

Brooten, D. A., Brown, L. P., Hollingsworth, A. O., Tanis, J. L., & Donlen, J. (1983). A comparison of four treatments to prevent and control breast pain and engorgement in non-nursing mothers. *Nursing Research, 32,* 225-229.

Deberry, P., Jefferies, L. P., & Light, M. (1975). Teaching cardiac patients to manage medications. *American Journal of Nursing, 75,* 2191-2193.

Ervin, C. T., Komaroff, A. L., Baranowski, K., & Pass, T. M. (1982). Behavioral factors and vaginitis. *The Nurse Practitioner: The American Journal of Primary Care, 7*(2), 20-21.

Friesen, L., & Stotts, N. A. (1984). Retention of basic cardiac life support content: the effect of two teaching methods. *Journal of Nursing Education, 23,* 184-191.

Grandjean, B. D., Bonjean, C. M., & Aiken, L. H. (1982). The effect of centralized decision-making on work satisfaction among nursing educators. *Research in Nursing and Health,* (5), 29-36.

Haber, L. C., Murphy, P. E., & Taylor, S. W. (1977). The effect of short-term group psychotherapy on the elderly. *The Canadian Journal of Psychiatric Nursing, 18,* 8-11.

Helton, M. C., Gordon, S. H., & Nunnery, S. L. (1980). The correlation between sleep deprivation and the intensive care unit syndrome. *Heart & Lung, 9,* 464-468.

Hoffman, M., Donckers, S., & Hauser, M. (1978). The effect of nursing intervention on stress factors perceived by patients in a coronary care unit. *Heart & Lung, 7,* 804-809.

Ingle, R. J., Burish, T. C., & Wallston, K. A. (1984). Conditionality of cancer chemotherapy patients. *Oncology Nursing Forum, 11* (4), 97-101.

Jackson, P. B., Bradham, R. F., & Burwell, H. K. (1978). Childcare in the hospital—a parent/staff partnership. *The American Journal of Maternal Child Nursing, 3* (2), 104-107.

Jordan, J., & Meckler, J. R. (1982). The relationship between life change events, social supports, and dysmenorrhea. *Research in Nursing and Health*, (5), 73-79.

Kathol, D. K. (1984). Anxiety in surgical patients' families. *Association of Operating Room Nurses Journal, 40* (1), 131-137.

Knafl, K. A. (1982). Parents' views of the response of siblings to a pediatric hospitalization. *Research in Nursing and Health*, (5), 13-20.

Lowrey, S. J., & Femea, P. L. (1984). The effect of in vitro use of heparin in blood transfusions during dialysis on dialyzer clotting. *American Association of Nephrology Nurses and Technicians Journal, 11* (2), 26-29.

McLendon, M. S., Fulk, C. H., & Starnes, D. C. (1982). Effectiveness of breast self-examination teaching to women of low socioeconomic class. *JOGN Nursing, 11* (1), 7-10.

Nelson, D. (1984). Nurse managed rehabilitation. *Nursing Management, 15* (3), 30-39.

O'Connell, K. A., Hamera, E. K., Knapp, T. M., Cassmeyer, V. L., Eaks, G. A., & Fox, M. A. (1984). Symptom use and self-regulation in type II diabetes. *Advances in Nursing Science, 6* (3), 19-28.

Osguthorpe, N., Roper, J., & Saunders, J. (1983). The effect of teaching on medication knowledge. *Western Journal of Nursing Research, 5*, 205-216.

Philbrick, M. (1984). Perceived importance of nursing and health care delivery issues. *The Journal of Continuing Education in Nursing, 15*, 205-208.

Pierce, S. F., & Thompson, D. (1976). Changing practice: by choice rather than chance. *The Journal of Nursing Administration, 6* (2), 13-19.

Putnam, S. T., McDonald, M. M., Miller, M. M., Dugan, S., & Logue, G. L. (1980). Home as a place to die. *American Journal of Nursing*, (*80*), 1451-1453.

Robarge, J. P., Reynolds, Z. B., & Groothius, J. R. (1982). Increased child abuse in families with twins. *Research in Nursing and Health*, (5), 199-203.

Schroeder, D. M., Cantor, M. M., & Kurth, S. W. (1981). Learning needs of the new graduate entering hospital nursing. *Nurse Educator, 6* (6), 10-17.

Scott, D. W. (1983). Anxiety, critical thinking and information processing during and after breast biopsy. *Nursing Research, 32*, 24-28.

Smith, S. P., Jepson, V., & Perloff, E. (1982). Attitudes of nursing care providers toward elderly patients. *Nursing and Health Care, 3*, 93-98.

Toney, L. (1983). The effects of holding the newborn at delivery on paternal bonding. *Nursing Research, 32*, 16-19.

Vik, A. G., & MacKay, R. C. (1982). How does the 12-hour shift affect patient care? *The Journal of Nursing Administration, 12* (1), 11-14.

Wagner, L., & Bye, M. G. (1979). Body image and patients experiencing alopecia as a result of cancer chemotherapy. *Cancer Nursing, 2*, 365-369.

Wall, D. T., & Gabriel, L. A. (1983). Alterations of taste in children with leukemia. *Cancer Nursing, 6,* 447-451.

Yeates, D. A., & Roberts, J. E. (1984). A comparison of two bearing-down techniques during the second stage of labor. *Journal of Nurse Midwifery, 29,* 3-11.

Chapter 14

Converting the Research Report into an Article

Every year hundreds of master's theses and dozens of dissertations are laid to rest on the shelves of nursing school libraries because their authors find it too difficult to cut 60–80 pages to 10. Here are some suggestions for doing just that—for pruning and shaping the original report and turning it into a brief, lucid, and publishable article. (Never submit the thesis itself for publication; it will be promptly rejected.) For the sake of brevity, the word "thesis" will be used from now on to stand for both types of reports. The guidelines will follow the format of the standard research article discussed in the previous chapter, and it will be referred to frequently. The previous chapter assumed that you were preparing a research article more or less from scratch, although you would undoubtedly have used parts of your original report, thesis, or dissertation. This chapter, in contrast, concentrates on *adapting* your original report into a publishable article. As such, there is bound to be some duplication between the two chapters, so choose accordingly.

In most research articles, the introduction is brief; the section describing the methods is somewhat longer; findings are presented succinctly and, depending on their complexity, may be brief or long; and, finally, the discussion of what it all means is usually substantial. Depending on the thrust of your article and the audience you envisage, you may want to alter the emphasis and expand or contract some of the parts. But whatever your thrust, the original thesis is unlikely to have the right proportions; indeed, the very opposite is more likely. This can be remedied with a little concentrated thinking, some good sharp scissors, and plenty of tape for rearranging and pasting. If you use a word processor instead of scissors, you can do the job more neatly. But however you edit, make a copy of your original before you begin, so you can look at it when you lose your way or think the old was better than the new.

Introduction and Literature Review

You'll need to cut more of the literature review than anything else. However, if the thesis did not begin with the review but with a brief introduction describing the problem and concluding with the purpose statement or an overview of the study methods, you can use that introductory section almost as is. Simply strengthen the middle of it with three or four paragraphs describing the studies closest to your own and pointing to shortcomings in those studies and gaps remaining in the research. The description can be condensed from the final pages of the literature review in the thesis. Omit the rest of the review.

If your thesis did not begin with a separate introductory section but plunged straight into the literature, the condensing is a little more complicated. First write an opening sentence or two, clearly identifying the problem or question studied. Then condense the last few pages of the literature review — the discussion of closely related studies — into a few paragraphs to establish the context for the study. Conclude with your purpose statement or overview.

If you tested any theoretical propositions or based your intervention on a theoretical model, the introduction should make that clear. Don't discuss theory in a separate section, however; incorporate it into the discussion of closely related work. Describe the theory *before* describing related empirical studies, if those were based on or tested the same theory. Discuss theory *after* those studies if you were the first to use the model or test the proposition.

If your study had no direct link to clearly identifiable theory, omit any mention of a theoretical framework. (More discussion of the use of theory is on pages 136–138.)

The introduction to the article should make the purpose, worth, and need for your study immediately clear. That is, it should tell why the study was necessary, what you intended to accomplish by it, and indirectly, why its outcomes are important. If those outcomes were not what you originally expected, the introduction can be a bit tricky. You need to point readers toward what you actually found instead of what you expected to find, and the thesis may not have done that. So as you condense, you may also need to alter the emphasis of the material. The best way to drop the right clues about where you're heading is to use the paragraphs discussing other studies to point to differing opinions or raise questions that your study will answer.

Methods

Articles don't have space for all the details about methods that go into a thesis or dissertation. Readers need only enough information to enable them to understand how you arrived at your findings and to evaluate their merit. But when you know everything about the study, it's hard to decide how much information is enough for others and to figure out which details they might need and which are nonessential. The temptation is to cut out nearly everything or leave everything as it is in the thesis. It's best to try for a middle ground, remembering that in a first draft, too much is better than too little; it's easier to condense or cut than to write more.

A good way to go about this is to read through the "Methods" section of your thesis, then put the thesis aside and write from memory, as if you were telling a story. Use this organization: first an overview of the methods, then the description of setting and sample, next the intervention, if applicable, and finally, measurements or data collection. If you do a first draft this way, you'll follow a logical organization and communicate the flow of the research without feeling tempted to put in every detail of the thesis. Then, once you have the basic information on paper, check it against the thesis to make sure you've included everything essential. Below are some guidelines on what to include in each part of the "Methods" section.

Overview and Hypotheses or Research Questions.   A one- or two-sentence overview or summary of the study methods begins this section, just as in the thesis; you can often lift it straight from the thesis. But check the statement against the concluding paragraph of your introductory section. If you have an overview there, don't repeat it here; if the purpose you gave there overlaps too much with the overview here, combine them into one statement, and put it either at the end of the introduction or at the beginning of "Methods."

You can list your hypotheses just as in the thesis, or you can add a sentence after the overview to tell readers more informally what you expected to find. The decision on whether to use formal hypotheses or not depends on the relation of your study to theory. If you presented an explicit theoretical framework in the introduction, it makes sense to state hypotheses; if you had no clear theoretical basis, simply communicate your expectations. And if you did not find what you expected, omit any mention of hypotheses or expectations, because they'll point readers in the wrong direction. Research questions can be stated explicitly if the article is formal; otherwise communicate them indirectly in the overview.

Definitions.   If your thesis contained a section titled "Definitions," it is best to get rid of it. When you use a term that your audience might not understand or give a special meaning to a commonly understood term, you should define the term the first time it appears in the narrative, not save the definition for a special section. Many of your definitions, however, are likely not to be definitions at all, but criteria for sample selection or descriptions of how you chose and used your variables; make those points clear in the appropriate places and don't repeat the information.

Setting and Sample.   Cut your description of setting and sample to the bare bones, leaving only enough information to prepare readers for any effects the sample selection may have on findings. Give the type of setting in a sentence—e.g., a 700-bed acute care hospital—then indicate directly or indirectly the manner of selecting the sample and list the criteria for inclusion in the study. If there was anything odd about your procedures for obtaining subjects, tell readers now, especially if you'll need to refer to this fact later in explaining findings. But don't make apologies for your sample, don't name names, and don't say how you got access to subjects. Do mention that you assured subjects of anonymity and confidentiality and that they signed a consent form.

Sometimes people describe sample characteristics at this point instead of in "Findings"; if you did that in the thesis, you may also want to do it in the article. However, the more important these characteristics are, the more useful it is to place them near the findings they might affect, so consider reorganizing.

Theses and dissertations generally provide a complete description of the sample; most of the information should be cut for the article. Describe only characteristics of major interest or influence, and do so in the narrative. Don't waste a table here, save it for more precious information, and don't choke the narrative with endless percentages.

Intervention.   The description of the intervention can often be lifted from the thesis without major changes, but if you gave a lot of detail there you may want to do some cutting and condensing. The amount of detail you need depends on the thrust of the article. If you are trying to convince readers that a new or complex treatment or program is both useful and feasible, you need to say how it's carried out. But if the intervention could be easily conceived by others, you don't need to give a lot of detail, just describe it generally. (On page 142 there's a brief description of a teaching program on seat belt usage for school aged children; that's an example of what I'm talking about.) If what mattered most about the study was not the intervention but the tool you used to assess its effectiveness or the theory on which it was based, don't spend a lot of time on the intervention itself.

Data Collection.   Measurement tools and the findings they produce are generally described in the same order. The standard organization is physiological measurements first, then scheduled observations, and finally questionnaires or interviews, thus moving from the more objective and precise to the more subjective and imprecise. But your most important findings may not have come from the most objective measurements and when you get to the "Findings" section, you'll probably want to give the most important information first. You may want to reorganize here to present the tools in the same order.

In the thesis, measurement tools are often only skimpily described; thesis writers tend to spend their time discussing validity and reliability studies and depend on an appendix to inform readers about the actual instruments. But there are no appendices in articles; in any case, you should always give readers enough information to enable them to anticipate the data you'll present. If your thesis did not do that, you may need to expand here, to communicate the flavor of your tools. (Suggestions for describing tools are given on pages 143–147.)

The main thing to remember is that the description of your instruments must prepare for all the findings you'll discuss later, but readers should not be led to expect information that will not be forthcoming. Depending on the focus of the article, you'll highlight some findings and cut or condense others, so you need to do the same with your tools: describe some parts in detail and cut out others. Then, when you've done a draft of both "Methods" and "Findings," look at them together to be sure they make a good fit.

If you used others' instruments, cut out the discussion of validity and reliability studies and simply note whether or not these have been established. If you developed the instrument yourself, describe any pilot tests or other efforts to establish validity and reliability, but keep the description brief.

Procedure.   When you come to this section of the thesis, look at its content together with your new draft of the rest of "Methods" and decide which of the research procedures can be omitted; then decide whether to incorporate the essential details into other descriptions or keep them in a separate section. For example, the procedures for acquiring subjects and ensuring that information about them will be kept confidential can usually be cut out, and your verbal or written assurances of confidentiality and anonymity can simply be mentioned in discussing the setting and sample. Similarly, some of the steps in taking subjects through the intervention can often be omitted and the rest integrated into the description of the intervention itself. But if the procedures for taking each subject through the research might be difficult to understand when spread around, it's best to keep them together and retain a separate section titled "Procedure."

If you decide to incorporate the material in other parts of the "Methods," make sure you include all the essential information and put it in the appropriate places. If you keep the material in a separate section, be sure to cut out irrelevant details and overlaps with other sections.

Data Analysis.   Thesis writers frequently explain in detail the technical operations they went through to analyze their data, sometimes even naming the statistical package used to prepare the data for testing and often describing particular tests of significance. For a journal article, however, you do not need to demonstrate that you understand statistics and have dealt appropriately with your data. Simply note what tests you used when you describe significance testing in "Findings."

Findings

Thesis findings often read like a computer printout perforated by verbal transitions. Everything is there just as it came out; there is no organization, nothing is highlighted or emphasized; it is all a monotonous plain. Thesis committees don't seem to mind, but readers of your article want only what really matters; they want what matters most to come first; and they want it with peaks and valleys. So you need to screen your material and perhaps reorganize.

Describing the Sample.   In an article, sample characteristics can be described in three places: (1) after the description of sample criteria and selection in "Methods," (2) at the beginning of "Findings," or (3) interspersed throughout "Findings," near the particular results they might be expected to affect.

The most logical place to describe the sample is at the beginning of "Findings," for sample characteristics are part of your findings and their description establishes a context for the rest of what you found. But that logic isn't always overriding. You may have described the sample in "Methods" in your thesis because it seemed to fit better there. It may still seem to fit better there in your article, especially if most of the sample characteristics were preset by your criteria for inclusion in the study, or the sample turned out to be skewed in some way, requiring explanation. In that case leave the description in "Methods."

If the sample characteristics are reasonably interesting and can be described briefly and straightforwardly, describe them at the beginning of "Findings." If your description was elsewhere in the thesis, it won't be hard to move it and it will make a nice introduction here. But if the description is of necessity long and complex, leave it in "Methods," for it will give your "Findings" section a dull, slow start and you don't want that. "Findings" should begin sharply, and impress readers immediately with the importance of the study outcomes.

If the sample turned out to be quite heterogeneous — a little of this and a little of that — give only the most basic information such as numbers and general types at the beginning of "Findings" and then bring up particular characteristics or groupings with the findings they affected (or you feared they might affect). Be sure to mention anything you controlled for, when you discuss the finding it was related to.

Describing the Findings.   It's a rare thesis that achieves the right organization and emphasis in the description of data, so be prepared to reshape the material in this section. First ask yourself what your most important findings were. If what mattered most was the expected, or the very opposite of the expected, clearly that's what you'll talk about first and most fully. If what really mattered, however, is something you discovered incidentally or through additional explorations, first briefly present the main answers to your original questions, no matter how muddy and disappointing; then move quickly on to the important findings. More detailed suggestions for organizing the description are on pages 148–150.

All major findings can be discussed before hypothesis testing, or you can present the data in relation to particular hypotheses. If you had several hypotheses, it's generally better to present all the findings, then discuss the hypotheses. If you had only one or two hypotheses, it works well to discuss data and hypotheses together.

Often thesis writers approach their major findings by first repeating verbatim the hypothesis at issue. Then they tell whether the hypothesis was supported and what tests were done to ascertain that; finally they describe the data. That's backwards. If you organized your findings in that way, turn them around for the article. First describe the data; or, if you think readers need an introduction, begin by restating the hypothesis or expected difference/association in the narrative, and then go on to describe the data. Next discuss differences or associations and tell whether they were significant. Name the test of significance used and give the p level in parentheses. If you explained the test in your thesis, cut that out. You do not need to describe a statistical maneuver in an article unless it would ordinarily be considered inappropriate for your data. (In such a case, point out the advantages for you of the technique used so that readers will understand why you chose it instead of some other.) If differences in the character of your groups might have accounted for a difference in outcome, indicate how you controlled for this, or else discuss it here as a limitation; don't save the problem for an arbitrary section called "Limitations."

You can conclude the discussion by noting that the hypothesis was supported, or you can leave that conclusion to readers. If your hypotheses were not supported, you need not mention them at all; in fact, it's better not to. Simply report what you found, note that it was unexpected, and say why you think it occurred. If you omit hypotheses here, however, you must go back and omit them in earlier sections, or rephrase them as expectations.

More detailed suggestions for presenting findings and tests of the hypotheses are on pages 151–152.

As you're reworking this section of the thesis, watch the length. If it goes on and on, you may need to consider cutting out some of your findings. Perhaps before you began, you decided to save some of the data for a second article; despite that, you still have too much. In that case, cut out some more, even though it may mean that you can't include all of your major findings. Step back and survey what you have, decide on a reasonable cutting off point, put some data aside for another article, and focus more sharply on what remains. Then redo your introduction and methods sections to fit the new focus.

If a hard look at the data convinces you that some of them

won't fit here, yet won't stand up alone to make another article, throw them out and don't worry about the loss. It's better for nursing and ultimately will be better for you to waste a few data than to insist on publishing every trivial fact you know.

Tables.   Articles rarely have space for more than two or three tables. How to decide which ones to keep, which to toss out? There are two ways to approach the problem. Before you begin the section on findings, look at the tables in the thesis, decide which two or three contain the vital information, and use them as the basis for putting this section together. Or don't look at your tables at all until you're into the narrative about findings; when you find yourself getting bogged down with numbers, turn to the thesis; there's doubtless a table to solve your problem. If you bog down and begin thinking about tables too often, see if you can combine two or three tables to save space, or prune the data enough to convey it in narrative form.

Don't write directly from a table or you'll find yourself just copying figures. Look at the table, then put it aside, and in the narrative highlight and interpret the main points. An illustrative table appears on page 150.

Comments and Anecdotal Data.   If you used comments and anecdotal data to enliven and explain your findings in the thesis, there's no reason to change that approach here. Just make sure that when you cut and condense findings, your comments fit what's left. If you saved your comments for the "Discussion" section in the thesis, you might want to move some of those up to "Findings" in the article. Comments are especially helpful along the way if you have complex data or a string of dry facts, for those can make the narrative very dull.

The use of anecdotal data depends on the audience you're aiming for and the tone of your writing. The more informal the article, the most helpful is the human touch that anecdotes convey. The more formal and starched your tone, the less appropriate are anecdotal data and the more you should confine your comments to logical explanations and speculations. See pages 152–155 for more discussion of comments and anecdotes.

Discussion

The discussion section is perhaps the most important part of an article, for it is this that takes readers beyond facts to the meanings they suggest, the questions they raise, the ideas they point to, and, ultimately, the uses they have for the world. Most readers remember a good article by its closing section; that's where they found the idea for a new study, realized the complexities of the theory they were planning to work with, or saw the possibility for better assessment or a new treatment or different arrangement.

The contents and organization of this section are described on pages 155–162. Basically, the discussion should show readers (1) the importance of the findings, (2) the limits to their generalizability, and (3) where applicable, their implications for research, theory, and practice, in that order. The concluding chapter of a thesis may contain this same material spread throughout several separate sections titled "Discussion," "Implications," "Limitations," "Suggestions for Further Research," and "Conclusions." In an article, these should be combined into one coherent statement or argument. The discussion may begin with a brief (two-sentence) review of the major findings, but it should not include a summary of the study: an opening abstract serves that purpose.

If the concluding section of your thesis fully explored the meanings and uses of your study, you'll need only to trim and shape for the article. Cut out summary and repetitions, combine separate sections to get the right order of points and make a flowing narrative, see that the focus is on what really matters, and cut out comments about findings that have been trimmed or downplayed.

If, however, you are one of those who wrote a perfunctory conclusion to the thesis, you must think through the implications of your work now. Essentially, you want to tell readers what the study means for them. The meanings may point in three directions: toward further research, theory development, and/or practice. Begin by making notes about what the study has to say in each of these areas, but don't make suggestions for further research that are in no way based on your study, don't tout the usefulness of a theory that proved useless for you, and remember what the real world is like before you propose putting an intervention into practice.

When you've thought through the possible meanings of your work, decide which of these is most important and appropriate to emphasize for your audience. If you are writing primarily for theorists or other researchers, you may want to focus on the study's implications for theory development, the questions it does not answer, or the possibilities it raises for further study. If you are writing for a broader audience of practicing nurses, you may want to concentrate on how the study findings can be used to improve patient care *now*.

In deciding what to highlight it is helpful to review your findings and look back at the introduction to the article. Those two sections together should help you clarify the thrust of your discussion. Then, once you've written this concluding section, examine all three sections together and see that they make a good fit. If you discuss theory in the opening section, for example, you must also deal with it in the conclusion. So if you decide while writing the article to shift your focus to practical uses, cut out the theoretical discussion in the introduction. Similarly, if your findings raise more questions than they answer, making it impractical to think of implementing your intervention, don't lead into the article by pointing to the practical importance of what you're doing.

Polishing and Refining

When you have a complete first draft of an article, put it beside the thesis and read the two together to be sure you haven't left out anything essential. Then put the thesis aside and concentrate on the article. Your task now is the task of every writer; you must revise and revise until, in a flowing narrative, everything from the first sentence on points toward your conclusions, the proportions along the way reflect the importance of each part to the whole, and everything hangs together to make a clear and cogent case. And if, in the process, you find that the suggestions given here cease to be useful, abandon them and go your own way, for ultimately the best guide is your own judgment.

Chapter 15

Writing an Article from the Data Sheets

Perhaps you did not have to write a research proposal in order to carry out your study, or you wrote only a very skimpy one, say for an institutional review board or for in-house funding. You may not have written a research report, either. So you'll be starting almost from scratch as you set out to report your study in an article. The outline on pages 122–123 will give you a guide to follow, and you may want to reread Part Three, chapters 12 and 13, to get a feel for what your article should contain. Below are some pointers for moving from the data to the article, with references to earlier chapters for detailed suggestions on how to organize and what to include.

While the discussion will take up each of the major sections of an article in the order in which they appear—"Introduction," "Methods," "Findings," "Discussion"—they needn't be written in that order. You may find it preferable to first write up some notes on the findings, then compose the "Methods" section, after that go back and complete "Findings," then write the "Introduction" and, finally, compose the "Discussion" section.

Or you can begin the article while you're still collecting data. That's a particularly good idea if your findings are looking good and the topic is important. In that case, write "Methods" first, then work on the "Introduction." Later, when you've analyzed the data and written up your findings, check all three sections to be sure they fit together. However you go about it, it's wise to get a first draft done as quickly as possible. You'll feel safer when it's all on paper, and that will make it easier to revise and reorganize as ruthlessly as you need to.

Introduction and Literature Review

If you wrote only a brief proposal or none at all and you wrote no research report, you may need to review the literature before you write this section, so that you can show how your study fits into the context of the work done to date and builds on that work. You won't be starting with nothing, however, for you undoubtedly did some work in the library before undertaking a study.

The process goes like this. You find a question you need to answer or a problem you must solve. Before trying to develop your own solution, you go to the literature to see whether someone else has solved the problem. If you discover a clear solution you do not need to invent one yourself or test its merit; hence there's no study. If you do not find a clear answer to your question, you may decide to do some research yourself; but you do it in the context of what's been done—the partial answers or solutions to date. You only need to articulate that context now.

You may already have notes from your review of the literature. If not, look back at the articles and pull out the relevant information; you also need to check recent journals in your selected area to see if other closely related studies have appeared since you started your research. If you find any recent studies that are troublingly close to yours, there are suggestions for dealing with them on pages 81-83.

When you have examined the literature, write a brief introduction that describes the problem, looks at the studies done before yours, and shows why your study was needed. Pages 133–138 give some advice on writing this introduction, with examples from published articles.

Methods

You don't start this section from scratch; you're reporting what you already know. To make it easier, before you begin, pull out the letter you sent the director of nursing or agency administrator explaining the study and requesting access to subjects, the criteria you used for including subjects in the study, the consent forms, the protocol you used for the intervention, hypotheses or research questions, your data collection sheets or questionnaires, and anything else you have on paper or can easily put on paper. Then, using these materials as a basis, outline the methods you used to carry out the study, following the outline given on pages 122–123. This will help you avoid organizational problems when you begin writing, and it will also give you a secure sense of what you have to say.

When you begin to write, it's helpful to think about what you did as if it were a story. Once upon a time you got a setting and sample, then you did something with or to your subjects, and then you measured some indicators of something. Write this section like a story, and it will be easy to read. Follow the guides given in Part Three, Chapter 13.

Be sure that you write what you actually did, not what you originally hoped to do and then found to be impossible. Make clear the criteria and method of selecting the sample and assigning people to groups (if you had groups). People often forget those details, but they are essential for judging the credibility of your findings. Also, describe your measurement instruments clearly enough so that readers will understand how you obtained the findings.

After you've drafted the meat of the section, go back and write the introductory overview of your methods. Have a couple of colleagues who know nothing of your study read your draft and tell you whether they understand what you did. If they do, you need add no more. If they don't, explain further wherever your methods seem unclear.

Findings

Preparing to Write. Before you even think about writing, organize your data. If you're working from computer printout, look through it and underline in red all those findings that seem interesting: a change in mean knowledge scores or attitudes or blood pressure or vital capacity, an association between age and incidence of confusional episodes, a surprising difference between nurses' and patients' views of the utility of intensive care—whatever strikes you.

It's useful to make a note about why a particular finding interests you. That will help you begin the process of thinking through the meanings of your findings, and it will then be easier to decide on the thrust of your article and the appropriate audience for it (see pages 127–130) for a discussion of how thrust and audience shape an article).

After you've underlined the interesting differences and associations, make some notes about how individual findings are related or can be grouped. To do that you may have to go through the printout repeatedly, for data come out in the order they were entered and related findings will not necessarily show up near each other.

When you have some notes about groups of findings, make a set of rough preliminary tables. It's much easier to write from tables than from computer printout, because the numbers are now ordered in a way to make their importance stand out. (See pages 103–104 for suggestions on constructing tables.) Decide which of the findings are most important and how you want to organize your description of them. Then you are ready to write.

If you are working with numbers but have not used a computer, group your figures into tables, pick out the differences and associations that are interesting, and make some notes about why they are important, then organize your description just as you would with data from the computer.

If you are working with information that cannot be transformed into numbers (for example, a series of open-ended interviews that produced widely varying responses), try to categorize or group related responses so that you can discuss classes of attitudes or views or situations. Then decide which are most common and important and organize your description on that basis.

Organizing the Description.   The standard organization of the "Findings" section is described fully on pages 148–152. Usually this section begins with a description of the sample, giving the final size and explaining any losses during the study. Next, the relevant sample characteristics are described, and then come the major findings. Hypothesis testing and exploratory analyses are presented after the data are described.

There are other ways to organize this section, however. Sometimes people describe sample characteristics and give the final sample size in the section on setting and sample in "Methods," instead of in "Findings." And when the study produced only a few major findings—for example, differences in outcomes between an experimental and comparison group—the description of the data is often combined with hypothesis testing (or significance testing if hypotheses are not stated formally). Choose the organization that best fits your study; the examples in Chapter 13 can serve as guides. But when guides don't seem to fit your data, follow your own judgment and common sense.

Comments and Anecdotal Data.   Sometimes researchers fear any data that do not arrive in numbers. But anecdotal data are also "data" and they can support or explain your numbers and enrich your description. Comments on the data are also important. If you have only a few major findings to present, you can save your comments for the concluding section of your article. If you have many smaller bits of information, however, comment as you go; otherwise, you have to repeat too much later to cue the reader in. Use the concluding section then to discuss the larger implications of your findings, taken all together.

Checking Findings Against Other Sections.   You may have more data than you can adequately describe in one article. If so, pick out all the information that is related to your main focus and that will add to the reader's understanding of your most important findings, and leave the rest for another day.

When you've completed this section, check back to make sure that the focus here is reflected in your earlier sections. In particular, make sure you have indicated in "Methods" how you got all the information you present here and have not led readers to expect data you do not deal with. If you did not prepare readers for some of the findings you discuss, go back and add to your description of measurement tools. Never discuss methods among the findings except in the case of additional, exploratory analyses done to figure out what your findings might mean.

Discussion

Gertrude Stein is reported to once have said, "A difference to be a difference must make a difference." It's a good motto—and especially useful to remember when you're writing the discussion section of a research article. Before you begin, ask yourself what difference it makes that you found a difference between x and y or an association between a and b. What are the meanings for others; why should they be interested? The answers to those questions will produce the heart of your concluding section and send readers away ready to adopt your new method of caring for terminal cancer patients, your strategy for improving clinical experiences of undergraduate nursing students, or a new conceptual model for looking at parental grief and guilt when a child dies.

Read through your findings and make notes about the meanings of what you found, then make notes about possible limits on their usefulness or generalizability. Next, jot down your ideas about how these limits might be overcome or otherwise dealt with. Then organize the discussion section following the outline on page 123.

To introduce readers to your thinking, begin by summarizing your major findings. But take only a sentence or two for the summary, even if it's tempting to run through all your main results again. (Going over familiar territory is easier than breaking new ground, but readers want constant discovery, not repetition.)

After you've restated your major findings, tell readers what those findings indicate. And if some of the findings seem to point in different directions, indicate your awareness of the apparent contradiction and try to clear it up. Note here any shortcomings in the study that might limit the generalizability or usefulness of the findings. Raise the questions a thoughtful reader might ask; answer them if you can; if you cannot, acknowledge that there are limitations and indicate how they might best be viewed and whether and how additional research might overcome them. Then suggest the implications for theory development, if appropriate, and the ways in which your findings can be used now in the practice of nursing. There are more detailed suggestions for writing the "Discussion" section, with examples, on pages 155–162.

When you have finished the draft of this section, lay your article aside for a few days, then come back and read it through from beginning to end, to see how it hangs together. Add information where you have been unclear, cut out nonessential facts, revise and edit, and conclude with a graceful, upbeat paragraph.

PART FOUR

Adjuncts to Preparing Research Proposals, Reports, and Articles

Inevitably, it seems, in preparing any book, there are always bits and pieces that don't fit appropriately in any chapter—or could go in any or all chapters. Consequently, for ready accessibility and to avoid duplication, these fragments are grouped together here in this final part of the book.

SECTION 1 FORMATS

Theses and Dissertations

Most universities publish guidelines for the preparation of theses and dissertations, giving information on format, typing, margins, corrections, and reproduction. A fairly standard format looks like this:

Standard Format

Title page, containing
1. the title of the thesis or dissertation
2. the candidate's name
3. a statement like this: A thesis (dissertation) submitted to the faculty of (university name) in partial fulfillment of the requirements for the degree of _____ in the Department (School) of _____.
4. the place and the date of acceptance of the manuscript by the committee
5. on the bottom right hand side, the words "Approved by" followed by a line for the signature of the advisor and two lines for signatures of readers (sometimes there is a separate approval page)

Abstract
   (usually not more than 100–150 words for a thesis and 300–350 for a dissertation, but may go as high as 600 words for the dissertation)

Table of contents

Acknowledgements

List of tables

Chapter I: Introduction and Review of the Literature

Chapter II: Methods

Chapter III: Findings

Chapter IV: Discussion

Bibliography (references)

Appendixes

Within the body of the work the format is flexible. The number of chapters, for example, may vary depending on the complexity of the material. The number and level of subheadings within chapters may also vary. Some authors begin each chapter with an introduction; some end each chapter with a summary. The best rule to follow is this: make it as easy as possible for readers to follow your argument, but submit them to no unnecessary repetition.

Articles

Like university guidelines for theses and dissertations, journal formats differ but the differences are not vast. Journals want a short but descriptive title and most also request a 100–200 word abstract. Every journal wants a short biographical sketch of the author—usually degrees and current position; some also want a photograph. A number of journals want a separate title sheet giving the title, author's name, degrees, and position. (Those journals usually do not want the author's name on every page of the text, to preserve anonymity in review; other journals are less concerned about this.)

Every journal wants typed, double-spaced copy on $8\frac{1}{2} \times 11$ paper with one- or one-and-a-half-inch margins. Some journals stipulate an original, along with several copies. Figures and tables should be prepared on separate sheets of paper, with their approximate location indicated in the text.

The length journals prefer varies, but 2500–3500 words (10–15 pages) is fairly standard. The reference system differs from journal to journal, as do headings and divisions of the article.

Basic information on preparation of the manuscript can usually be found at the bottom of the journal's masthead page. More complete guidelines for authors are usually sent in response to a query letter, or simply call and ask for a copy. (In fact, it's a good idea to collect a file of these guidelines as an aid to publication.) Always check a recent issue of the journal to which you plan to submit your article before typing the final copy, to be sure that you're consistent with other articles there.

SECTION 2   REFERENCES

Keeping and Using References

Most research texts include suggestions on how to make notes and keep track of your references. People's habits range from the

188 Adjuncts to Preparation

nearly haphazard to the compulsively complex. With references, it is better to err on the side of compulsion. Nearly everyone can recall reading a useful article but losing the reference and then spending frustrating hours trying to relocate the material. Some can also remember reading a useless article over and over because they made no notes and forgot it was useless.

It's a good idea to make notes, with complete reference information, about everything you read that's remotely related to possible research or articles. The notes need only indicate what struck you as interesting or possibly useful for later reference. Develop at least a rudimentary filing system to keep track of what you have.

When you're preparing a proposal and making a focused review of the literature, obviously you need fuller notes on important works. As a rule of thumb, however, if an article seems important enough to summarize, it's usually more efficient to photocopy it.

As you write a proposal, thesis, or article, you'll have to decide what to reference and what not to reference. Worry only about the gray area where you feel uneasy and slightly guilty. It's unnecessary to reference everything in your head. All of us know a fair amount that we've learned on our own, from experience and observation, from the talk of others, from idle moments of imagining life. We also know a lot that's general information, widely known and belonging to no one. Most of the time you know very well when the point you're making is your own, and you also know when it's general information. You don't need to search for references for such points; there's such a thing as overdoing it (and thereby looking childish and insecure).

You also know when the idea or information you're presenting comes from a particular author or authors. Always reference such points. Difficulty occurs only when you've integrated others' ideas, theories, or data so thoroughly that you're not quite sure whether something is yours or theirs. When you feel that kind of uncertainty, check the reference. It's better in such cases to overcite than undercite. But in general, your conscience will guide you effectively on these points.

Reference Citations

There are a number of systems for reference citations, but the most rational and the easiest to use is the system of the American Psychological Association (APA), described in full detail in the APA's *Publication Manual,* third edition, 1983. The APA manual should be on your desk whenever you write, for its usefulness extends well beyond references, but here we'll talk only about those.

Briefly, the system is as follows. When you refer to a work in the text, give the author's last name and the date of publication of the work being cited in parentheses, thus: (Jones, 1980). If you use a direct quote, give the page number after the date. If the work has two authors, give both names, separated by an ampersand (&), each time you refer to the work, thus: (Jordan & Meckler, 1982). If the work has more than two authors and fewer than six, list them all the first time you refer to the work but after that give only the first author's name and "et al.," which means "and others," thus: (Smith et al., 1980). If the work has six or more authors, use *et al.* the first time.

If you refer to more than one work by the same author at the same point in your text, give the dates of the works in chronological order, separated by commas: (Jones, 1980, 1981, 1982). If two of the works are in the same year, give one of them an "a" and one a "b," and so on: (Jones, 1981a, 1981b).

If you are referring to works by different authors at one point in the text, arrange them alphabetically by the authors' last names, and separate the works by semicolons, thus: (Jones, 1980; Smith, 1982).

Usually you put the citation at the end of a sentence. For example, "Few of the elderly receive treatment for depression (Jones, 1970)." If it seems more appropriate, however, put the citation elsewhere in the sentence, thus: "One study (Jones, 1970) found that many women did not know how to do breast self-examination." And if you mention the author's name in the sentence proper, give only the year of publication in parentheses, right after the author's name—for example, "Jordan and Meckler (1982) concluded that the small correlations they found between life change events and dysmenorrhea were statistically significant because of large sample size."

With the APA system, references are listed at the end of the proposal or report or article in alphabetical order, regardless of the order in which they appear in the text. For journal articles, the author's last name appears first, followed by first and middle initials, then (in parentheses) the year of publication. The article title follows, with only the first word capitalized. Then comes the full name of the journal, underlined and with all major words capitalized; the volume number, underlined; and the inclusive pages, last. For books, the same general principles are followed, except that the title of the book is italicized (underlined) and the place of publication comes next, separated by a colon from the publisher's name.

The APA Manual gives countless examples of how to set up articles, books, and documents, with various combinations of authors or no authors. People often find that among all these examples the only one missing is the one they need. When that happens, just follow the example that seems nearest to yours and don't worry.

What makes the APA system so easy to work with is the use of names in the citations in the text. With other systems, when you move paragraphs around or even sentences, you run the risk of getting your references confused. Number 1 is now where number 6 was and you must remember to switch all numbers or all is lost. With the APA system you don't have to worry; the necessary information goes with the sentence or paragraph when it moves. The alphabetical listing at the end means you don't have to move things around there, either.

The APA system is also easy on readers, who discover what authors you're referring to as they read instead of having to go to your reference list to get the information. It's sensible to use this system for everything you write because the more you use it, the easier it is to remember all the tiresome details. Here are a few to watch for:

When you give a reference citation at the end of a sentence, always put it before the period, thus: (Jones, 1980). The parenthetical citation is a part of the sentence, not information to dangle between sentences.

When you say "Jones et al.," never put a comma after Jones.

You would never write, "Jones, and others went to the beach." So don't write "Jones, and others" here.

Never put a period after *et*; it is not an abbreviation but a word meaning "and." Always put a period after *al.*, which is an abbreviation for *alia*, meaning "others."

Include in your reference list only those authors you have cited in the text. And remember that in the reference list, the year of publication follows the author's name, coming before the title of the work.

Some journals use an author-date system of citing references in the text but do not put a comma between author and date, thus: (Bordeaux 1985). And many journals use a numbering system for citing references—in part because numbers take up much less space than names and dates. The reference number may be given in parentheses, inside the period at the end of the sentence, thus: (1). Or the number may be written as a superscript after the period, thus: .[1] A few journals put the reference number after the period, in brackets: .[1]

With numbering systems, references are usually listed at the end of the article in the order in which they were cited in the text, rather than alphabetically. Different journals set up the references in different ways.

When you are ready to publish an article, always check the journal to which you are submitting it and use that journal's reference system. It's easy to switch from APA style to another. Reference systems are like Romance languages: When you get the hang of one, the others aren't so hard to figure out. Your only enemy is carelessness.

SECTION 3 APPENDIXES

Lengthy materials that are not necessary for clarity but provide supporting evidence for statements made in a narrative are usually placed in an appendix. If put in the body of the work they would clutter up the narrative and interrupt the flow. Readers who want to check the accuracy or appropriateness of narrative statements are directed to the complete supporting documents in the appendix. For example, in a proposal, thesis, or dissertation you inform readers that you have explained your study to potential subjects and included only those people who signed a consent form. It would waste space and be an intrusion, however, to include the explanation and consent form in the narrative. Furthermore, they are not necessary to make the point. Therefore, you put these in an appendix, to show interested readers that you adequately explained the study and that the consent the subjects gave was *informed* consent.

Materials commonly included in the appendixes of research proposals, theses, dissertations, and reports are the explanation of the study to persons who granted access to subjects, the explanation of the study given to potential subjects, the consent form, complete protocol for the intervention, copies of all data collection instruments, and additional tables. Grant proposals often also include preliminary data or assessments, biographical sketches and job descriptions of project personnel, description of available resources, supporting letters, and information on contractual or collaborative arrangements.

Related materials should be grouped together and each set put in a separate appendix. For example, all materials related to acquisition of subjects would be in one appendix, and all data collection instruments in another. Each appendix is given a number or letter and a title, and a separate title page. For example, "Appendix C" might be titled "Assessment Survey."

SECTION 4   ABSTRACTS

When you submit a thesis or dissertation to the graduate school, an abstract must accompany it. If you want to present your research at conferences or symposia, you must send an abstract of the study to a selection committee. Most funding agencies require an abstract to precede a grant proposal, and many journals want an abstract to accompany articles submitted. Clearly it is important to know how to write an abstract.

There are two basic types of abstracts: descriptive and informative. The descriptive abstract, like a table of contents, describes the contents of a study or article, rather like this:

A brief overview of the study design is presented, and findings from Phase I of the study are discussed. The author draws conclusions for critical care nursing practice.

Rarely will you need to write that kind of abstract, although informative abstracts occasionally veer toward it, especially in presenting complex conclusions.

The informative abstract is what you'll be writing for your thesis or dissertation, for research conferences, and for journals. This abstract presents the purpose, explains the study methods, and summarizes findings and (sometimes) conclusions. It is essentially a synopsis of the study, like this one written to precede the article on "Parents and the Sexuality of Preschool Children" (Aquilino & Ely, 1985) quoted in Part Three, Chapter 13:

Eighty-one parents with preschool children were surveyed regarding the sexual activity and curiosity of 3 to 5 year olds. Positive relationships were found between parents' knowledge, responses, and comfort related to preschool sexuality. Discussions revealed that even knowledgeable parents lacked confidence in their abilities to deal with their child's sexuality.

Here's a longer and fuller abstract, from Jordan & Meckler, 1982, quoted in Part Three, Chapter 13:

A survey of 156 female undergraduate nursing students was conducted to determine the relationship between life change events and dysmenorrhea and the mediating effects of social supports on this relationship. Data were collected using the Anderson College Schedule of Recent Experience (subjects estimated personal readjustment to life changes), the Moos Menstrual Distress Questionnaire, and a social support index constructed by the authors. Correlations were obtained separately for high and low social support groups; these ranged from .19 to .62 and were significant ($p < .05$) for both groups. Presence or absence of a confidant was the most discriminating social support dimension ($r = .32$ for those with a confidant and .62 for those without). For subjects using oral contraceptives there was no relationship between life change and dysmenorrhea, while users of other contraceptives showed a significant positive relationship ($p < .05$). Life change and social supports together accounted for only 16% of the variance in menstrual distress scores. Methodological difficulties in using the life change and social support tools were identified.

In writing an abstract, the problem is how to give a clear and reasonably complete view of a study in a very few words. The maximum number of words permitted varies considerably—from a brief 50 to 75 words for some journals, to a single- or double-spaced page or page and a half for most research conferences, to a maximum of 600 words (two pages double spaced) for *Dissertation Abstracts*. The variations in length reflect the different uses of abstracts. The journal reader who sees an abstract at the head of the article needs only enough information to decide whether or not to read the article. A committee that must decide whether to select a study for presentation at a conference needs considerably more detail. And researchers combing *Dissertation Abstracts* for useful work in their area need fairly complete information.

The more space you have, the easier it is to abstract, obviously. It's also easier to abstract a proposal than a completed study, because there's less to describe. But the difficulties of abstracting are often exaggerated. This is a skill that can easily be acquired; it just takes time and a little thought. One way to learn is to begin abstracting journal articles that you particularly like. It's easier to summarize other people's work than your own, and you'll get the hang of abstracting while making useful notes for your reference file.

Most informative abstracts include a statement of the problem and the purpose of the study, information on subjects, the method of carrying out the intervention (if applicable), data collection techniques and instruments, procedures for analysis (if out of the ordinary), a summary of major findings, and conclusions emanating from the findings. Thus, all the parts of an article, proposed presentation, thesis, or dissertation are represented in the abstract except the literature review. That should be summarized only if you have space to spare. People sometimes leave out conclusions and applications, but they may be important in helping readers interpret and assess the importance of findings. If the study was based on a particular theoretical framework or tested theoretical propositions, that too is important to say.

Grant Writing for Health Professionals by Harry A. Sultz and Frances S. Sherwin has very useful suggestions for writing the abstract that must accompany a grant proposal. The *Publication Manual of the American Psychological Association* tells what to include in the abstract of an article or paper for presentation. *Research in Nursing* by Holly Skodol Wilson includes a guide for preparing abstracts. And Ellen O. Fuller's article, "Preparing an Abstract of a Nursing Study," in the September/October 1983 issue of *Nursing Research* gives very helpful examples and explains why some information is included in the abstract and some is excluded.

Here are a few suggestions for writing a medium-length abstract such as you might submit to a graduate school or a selection committee for a research conference. (Don't worry about length until you have completed a draft.)

First identify the problem and the study purpose; if the study was directly based on or tested theory, describe the theory and make clear the study's relation to it. If you cannot do so in two sentences at most, the connection to theory may not be direct enough to mention.

If you are abstracting a thesis or dissertation, you can often use the opening sentence of the introductory material as a basis for describing the problem, and you may be able to do no more than copy the purpose statement with which you concluded the literature review. If the purpose statement makes the problem sufficiently clear, omit the problem description; there's not room in an abstract to say the same thing twice, even in different words.

The overview of the study methods at the end of the literature review or at the beginning of the methods chapter serves as a framework for describing methods in the abstract, and it sometimes communicates the purpose of the study with enough clarity to make a purpose statement inessential.

Omit hypotheses and research questions; there's not room for everything and it's more important to tell what you did than what you were looking for. Give the sample size and method of selection, a sentence about the intervention if the study included one, and a list of all data collection instruments and techniques. (A list of these latter often introduces the section in the thesis titled "Data Collection" or "Variables and Their Measurement"; just copy it.)

Next present major findings, indicate whether you found any statistically significant differences or associations, and give the significance level in parentheses. Many theses and dissertations begin the concluding chapter with a summary of major findings;

use that summary as a basis for your description here. Or, if you're working from computer printout or tables, list what you consider to be the most important findings and turn these into two or three sentences. Finally, point out the implications of your findings—for theory if you mentioned theory earlier in the abstract, and for practice. Don't get into limitations or suggestions for further research.

When you have written a draft of the abstract, check it for completeness and clarity, and then see whether your word count is over the limit. If you are close to the requirements you can usually come within the maximum by pruning every bit of repetition, turning clauses into phrases, cutting out little words like "the" and "an," and otherwise tightening up the writing. If you are well over the maximum, you will probably have to omit some information. Try combining problem and purpose, leaving out further details of methods, and in the last resort cutting out the conclusions. Keep the emphasis on findings. Remember what Fuller says: "An abstract is a summary of the major findings of a study accompanied by enough description of the design and methods to allow the informed reader to put the results in perspective" (1983, p. 317).

SECTION 5 RESEARCH PRESENTATIONS

Presenting your research at conferences and symposia is not only a good way to begin getting your results out to people who can use them, but it is also a good way to move towards writing an article. Once you've organized your study results for a presentation, it's not hard to go a step further and turn the speech into an article. And the questions and comments you get from an audience will help you shape the article and refine and clarify your interpretation of the data.

The organization of a research presentation is similar to that of an article (see Part Three), but the emphasis differs. The time for a presentation is always limited, usually to no more than 10 or 15 minutes, and you want to use that time on what matters most. Therefore, it's wise to shorten the introduction and literature review even further than you would for an article, and omit the details of methods. Concentrate on the findings and your interpretation of them.

Below are a few suggestions for organizing each part of the presentation and then some comments about pitfalls to avoid, whether you are reading a paper or talking from notes and memory. Either way it is very helpful to use transparencies (or slides), handouts, or both. The visual representations help audiences understand complexities that are difficult to grasp when only hearing them. Don't overdo the use of visual aids however. Audiences are not simple minded and should not be treated as if they can grasp nothing that doesn't come in a picture.

An abstract and tables make particularly useful handouts, since they allow the audience to look back, to review. Other complex information can be given in transparencies or slides alone. Although they require more preparation, it is easier to use slides, because then you don't have to interrupt your thoughts to remove one and insert another (and you don't have to worry about putting them in the projector upside down).

The Introduction

Begin by giving the purpose of the study; don't build up to it as you might in an article. Listeners need to get a sense of what this is about right away. Make the literature review even briefer than you would for an article, and as you describe the work already done on your problem or question, avoid authors' names unless they are crucial; they will distract listeners from the more important information. As you conclude the introductory remarks, it's useful to repeat the study purpose to prepare the audience for methods.

Methods

Give an overview of the study just as for an article; if the design is at all complex, use a transparency or slide to help the audience grasp its various aspects. The content of hypotheses and research questions should be conveyed, but less formally than in an article. Tell how you got your sample, and if the criteria for inclusion in the study were complex, list them on a transparency or slide. Briefly describe the intervention if the study included one, then name the data collection instruments and say what they measured. Omit the details and don't mention validity and reliability at all unless your emphasis was on instrument development or your findings call into question the usefulness of your instruments. Keep the methods section short.

Results and Discussion

Your presentation should emphasize results and discussion, but don't overwhelm the audience. Describe your main findings in a general way and use slides for the numbers. Begin by describing the sample, but do that quickly, just giving highlights. Concentrate on the most important findings of the study and make sure the audience understands their relevance; omit minor findings or exploratory analyses. (But take a copy of all your tables with you, so that if questioned about further analyses you will have the information at hand.)

If you found significant differences or associations, point them out. Don't describe the statistics, however, unless they were new or different or might seem on first hearing to be inappropriate for your data.

Comment on the meaning of the findings as you present them. If you wait until a later discussion section to comment, the audience won't remember the data and you'll waste time repeating information. Conclude with a discussion of overall meanings and implications for nursing theory, research, and practice.

Preparing for the Presentation

In preparing your talk, the first decision you must make is whether to read the paper or talk from notes and/or memory.

While most audiences prefer a talk, many presenters prefer to read their papers, and at the big scholarly meetings in most disciplines almost no one speaks informally. You should do what seems most comfortable for you. There are dangers either way, but you can avoid them if you plan.

If you read your paper, two things to watch out for are droning on without expression or warmth and overwhelming the audience with so much detail they get no sense of the whole. A third danger is losing your place in the paper when you look up at the audience, so that you have to fumble around to find the next sentence.

Type the paper in all capital letters (they're much easier to read than upper and lower case letters), and triple space. That will make it easier to keep your place. Practice reading the paper over and over—preferably, before a mirror—until you are extremely familiar with it and feel free to look up from time to time and even to ad lib a bit. Eye contact keeps the audience paying attention, and a little informality helps to win them over. Before you go to the conference, read the paper to a few of your colleagues and ask them to suggest ways to make the content clearer and the delivery more lively. Check your time also. You don't want to be stopped by a time keeper just as you arrive at the main points.

If you decide to talk from memory, the major dangers are that you will omit basic information or rush past important points, then circle back to them, confusing the audience. You can even lose your way completely, forgetting the logic of your study. As a backup for memory, use a series of slides or transparencies and type the major points you want to make on 6×8 cards, in all caps and triple spaced. Don't use smaller cards or you'll fumble with them. Practice your talk until you are entirely comfortable with it, then ask your colleagues to listen, make suggestions, and time the presentation.

When you are comfortable with the talk or the paper, there is only one further danger: the question and answer session. Take any additional information you think might be asked for and prepare for questions and comments. When they come, don't be defensive. Be gracious about comments, answer all the questions you can, and when you don't know the answer, admit it. The best rule for a discussion session is be unfailingly polite.

Note: Don't submit your presentation, triple spaced and typed all in capitals, to a journal for consideration. It's hard to take in the sense of such a document, it presents a ferocious task of editing, and it's obvious you're trying to kill two birds with one stone. At least, retype it.

SECTION 6 THE QUERY LETTER

A query letter is a letter to the editor of a journal inquiring about interest in reviewing an article for possible publication. If you know which journal you want to send your article to and you're sure it's appropriate for that journal, there's no point in writing a query letter (unless the journal requires it, and a few do). You might as well send the article and take your chances. But often an article that seems appropriate for a particular journal isn't. In a survey of journal editors a few years ago, McCloskey and Swanson (1982) found that a common reason for rejecting articles was that the subject matter was not appropriate for the journal's audience. That same article is an excellent description of nursing and other health care journals. Another article by the same authors (Swanson and McCloskey, 1982) describes the review process in detail and indicates which nursing journals are refereed. Both articles are important resources for authors.

Since you can (ethically) submit your article for consideration to only one journal at a time and the review process takes two or three months at least (and often much longer), you waste a lot of time when you send an article to the wrong journal. So if you're not entirely sure where to send it, it's useful to query all the journals you think might be interested. You'll get a quick response from the editor or a staff member (usually within two or three weeks), telling you whether or not the journal is interested in seeing your article. Then you can eliminate those journals with no interest. (Sometimes, however, you simply get a form letter saying, "Send it along," which doesn't help you much.)

Sometimes the journal to which you plan to submit your article will have already accepted an article on that topic, though it has not yet appeared. The editor is unlikely to accept another on the subject right away, because readers want variety. If you write a query letter, you'll discover that, though appropriate, your article is unlikely to be accepted or, if accepted, may have to wait a year or more to be published.

There are other advantages to writing query letters. Journal editors who respond positively usually send along the journal's guidelines for authors, which give instructions on format and often add suggestions on style and organization. Sometimes editors give a bit of personal advice, tell you that they're interested in a particular slant, or warn that while they're willing to review the article their interest in the topic is limited. That information helps you decide on which journal to send the article.

Most nursing journals like to see a query letter before receiving the article. Many other health and health-related journals do not; they say a query doesn't give them enough information to make a decision so they'd rather see the article. Swanson and McCloskey (1982) tell which journals do and which do not want a letter.

A query letter should not be longer than a page. It ought to tell the editor what the article is about, why the topic is important, and what your credentials are for writing the article. You can indicate the importance of the topic indirectly in an opening sentence or two, pointing to the frequency or severity of the problem your study treats or the importance of the question it answers. If you note that you sought an answer to the question or solution to the problem and, finding none, undertook a study, you'll also indirectly establish your credentials and prepare for the description of your article. You may need to add that you've been working in this area for several years, to shore up your credentials. It's inadvisable, however, to point out that the research was done as part of the requirements for a master's or doctoral degree; then editors fear that you'll ship them the thesis or dissertation as is. Just give your degrees after your name. When the article is accepted, you can supply the details.

Next, write a one-paragraph summary of the study and indicate where the emphasis of the article lies—whether on methodological issues, the startling or controversial nature of the findings or their clinical significance, the ease with which your intervention can be used in a variety of settings, or the implications of your work for theory. Knowing the thrust of your article will help the editor decide whether it is suitable for the journal's audience.

If you have written an abstract of your study, you can work

from that. But an abstract rarely highlights anything and it gives no clues as to your normal writing style, so it's better not to copy it but just use it as a basis for writing the summary.

Conclude by saying that if the editor is interested you would like to submit the article for review (or "for possible publication"). This lets the editor know that you know a positive response to a query letter guarantees only consideration, not publication.

A few final words of advice. Don't type a general letter and insert a different address at the top for each journal you're querying (unless you're using a word processor). Editors want to be approached individually, not en masse. And check the masthead of a recent issue of each journal to be sure you know who the current editor is. There's hardly a worse insult than a letter addressed to a previous editor; that says you aren't reading the journal or even bothering to check it. Try to look like a reader even if you aren't.

SECTION 7 ORGANIZATION OF A GRANT PROPOSAL

The most important rule for writing a grant proposal is to follow the funding agency's guidelines to the letter. Often they seem to encourage repetition; sometimes they appear illogical or even incomprehensible. But like the instructions for completing your income tax return, these guidelines have been carefully designed and worded and it's important to follow them. The following is a fairly standard outline for a grant proposal.

Grant Proposal Format

Abstract
Specific aims (purposes and hypotheses or research questions)
Significance of the proposed research
Preliminary work (or pilot studies, or relevant experience of the principal investigator)

Experimental design and methods
  Overview of the study, with purposes, hypotheses, and/or
    research questions
  Setting
  Population to be studied, with sampling method, criteria
    for inclusion, expected size of sample, assignment to
    groups, and protection of human subjects
  Intervention protocol, if applicable
  Data collection instruments and procedures
  Time line for carrying out the study
  Analyses planned
References
Appendixes

In proposals to federal agencies, there are a number of additional sections. The abstract is followed by a budget, with justifications for all expenditures planned; biographical sketches of the principal investigator and all co-investigators; information on any other grant support of the investigators, or proposals pending review; and a description of the resources available to the investigators such as laboratories, clinical facilities, and computer capabilities. Then comes the body of the proposal, which is organized just as in the outline given above.

After the body of the proposal there is a section on human subjects (or vertebrate animals). It must contain a letter from an institutional review board indicating that the research is exempt from review, or a letter of approval indicating that the board has reviewed the proposal and found that the research is in compliance with federal regulations on the protection of the rights of human subjects. If the research is not exempt, this section must describe in detail subject recruitment procedures, consent procedures, possible risks and benefits to subjects, steps to be taken to minimize any risks, and confidentiality safeguards.

Next comes a list of consultants, with a curriculum vitae for each, and a description of any consortium or co-sponsorship arrangements. References and appendixes are last. The appendixes should contain all measurement instruments/protocols, relevant publications by investigators (especially the principal investigator), and any other materials that might help reviewers assess the adequacy of the methods or the competence of the investigators.

The outline used for proposals to Sigma Theta Tau, the outline of the American Nurses' Foundation, and the outlines of most private foundations are quite similar to the one given here, with some additional sections similar to those required by federal agencies. At first glance they seem very different from the outline for a thesis or dissertation proposal given in Part One, but the differences are in fact not great. In the body of the proposal it's mostly a matter of how you arrange the sections; the information that must be conveyed is much the same. *Grant Writing for Health Professionals* by Harry A. Sultz and Frances S. Sherwin is an invaluable resource for writing all sections of a proposal.

Following are a few suggestions for organizing the abstract and the sections on specific aims, significance, and preliminary work. The section on experimental design and methods is organized exactly as in a thesis or dissertation proposal.

Abstract

The abstract for a grant proposal is similar to the short introduction that often begins a thesis or dissertation proposal, except that it goes further and summarizes the proposed methods. First indicate the significance of the problem or question to be studied, point out the gaps or shortcomings in the work done to date on the problem, and give the purpose of the study, with hypotheses or research questions. Then give a clear overview of the study methods, indicating major variables, sampling method, intervention (if applicable), and data collection instruments.

Space is always limited, but some reviewers may read only the abstract, not the body of the proposal; it's wise, therefore, to use all the space you're allowed and make a strong case for the significance of the problem, the utility of the study, and the adequacy of the methods you're proposing.

Specific Aims

Specific aims should begin with a brief description of the problem and the gaps or shortcomings in the work done to date on it. This establishes the rationale for the study, its justification. Then give the long-term or overall goal (or long-range objective) of the proposed research and next, the specific aims, purposes, or objectives. Finally, list the study hypotheses or research questions.

The terms "goals," "purposes," "aims," and "objectives" overlap considerably. "Goals" is usually preferred to point out the ultimate utility of the research. The other three terms are almost synonymous. Whether you call them aims, purposes, or objectives, it's important to say clearly what the research is intended to accomplish. State your aims in such a way that readers will see that they are attainable and measurable. (How they are to be attained is not part of this section, but belongs in methods.)

The section on specific aims is somewhat like the concluding paragraphs of the literature review chapter of a thesis or dissertation proposal, which pull together the work done to date and give the purpose of the proposed study, its usefulness for nursing, and the study hypotheses. Purposes and hypotheses are stated exactly as in any other proposal.

Significance

The section on significance is very similar to the literature review of a thesis or dissertation proposal except that it is very condensed and must make explicit the importance of the proposed research. Begin by describing the problem or question and indicating its importance, spread, seriousness, or relation to serious problems. Then review the work already done on the problem, both theoretical and empirical. It is crucial to show how the proposed study is related to ongoing research in the discipline, so this review should describe work currently underway. That seems unreasonable; how is one to know? It isn't always easy. You may have to telephone people who've done important work in the field to see what they're doing now or ask federal agencies or foundations what research in the area they're currently funding. It is important to take the trouble to find out what is being done because this shows reviewers that you are aware of the most current work and helps to establish your credibility.

In the final paragraphs of this section, discuss the study you are proposing and show how it will contribute to solving the problem or answering the question and what the practical (or theoretical) benefits will be. In other words, show reviewers why the research is important. It is helpful to conclude with specific purposes because while that may overlap with the preceding section, the aims are the logical way to tie this whole discussion of significance together.

Preliminary Work

If the proposed study will build on or continue an earlier study of yours, report the earlier work here. Describe the methods and the findings and indicate how they laid the foundation for what you are now proposing. Any publications from the earlier study should be included in the appendixes.

If you have done a pilot study to refine your intervention or test your data collection instruments or procedures, report that work here just as you would report an earlier study. Give methods and findings and indicate how they support the feasibility and utility of the proposed study and what changes or refinements in the intervention or data collection instruments you have made.

If you have nothing preliminary to report, discuss any experience of the principal investigator that might be relevant to this research and that will help to establish that person's competence.

Experimental Design and Methods

The methods section is organized just as in a thesis or dissertation proposal. But in a couple of areas, additional information is necessary. In describing the study population and sampling procedure, for example, you must indicate how you will ensure that you have a sufficient sample. Describe your experience in and plans for recruiting and maintaining the study population and any plans you have for dealing with losses in that population.

In describing the intervention, data collection instruments and procedures, and plans for analysis, discuss any possible alternative approaches and explain why you chose one approach over another.

And finally, the data analysis section needs to be more complete than is usual in a thesis or dissertation proposal. Think through all the data you will collect and describe exactly what you will do with it.

SECTION 8   AIDS TO WRITING

There are many books about writing and a number of them are very helpful. Some are even quite enjoyable to read. But reading about writing is no substitute for writing, though it can be a tempting evasion. If you keep only a few books on the subject handy, you can avoid temptation and still find answers to most of your questions.

First on your list should be a good college-level dictionary. Use it whenever you have the slightest doubt about a spelling or the meaning of a word, so that you don't write subtle as "suttle" or say "in lieu of" when you mean "in view of." (A thesaurus or dictionary of synonyms will help you avoid using the same word over and over and can sometimes help you find the precise word you're looking for.)

A good freshman English handbook is also a useful reference, though I wouldn't recommend reading one from start to finish. Most have detailed tables of contents and excellent indexes, so that it's easy to find the answer to questions about grammar, punctuation, mechanics, and the organization of larger elements in a paper. Good handbooks include *The Writer's Companion* by William H. Roberts (in paperback), *The Brief English Handbook* by Edward A. Dorman and Charles W. Dawe (also in paperback), the *New English Handbook* by Hans P. Guth, *Handbook for Writers* by Glenn Leggett, C. David Mead, and William Charvat, and *A Short Guide to English Composition* by William A. McQueen (paperback).

Two grammar books that I've found both sensible and entertaining are *The Elements of Style* (third edition) by William Strunk, Jr., and E. B. White, and *The Handbook of Good English* by Edward D. Johnson. Both are in paperback. *The Elements of Style* contains eleven elementary rules of usage, eleven elementary principles of composition, a list of commonly misused words and expressions, and a section called "An Approach to Style (with a List of Reminders)." It is eminently readable and if you stay with these elementary rules and reminders, your writing cannot go far wrong.

The Handbook of Good English is in four parts: grammar, punctuation, miscellaneous mechanics, and diction and composition. The entries are clear (and often amusing) paragraphs explaining the whys of rules and also giving instances when it's better not to follow them—at least not slavishly. For example, the entry on the passive voice explains that while it can be distracting and cumbersome, the passive has its uses, including "the trouble-saving passive," "the passive to emphasize the agent," and "the pussyfooting passive."

A standard research text like *Nursing Research: Principles & Methods*, by Denise Polit and Bernadette Hungler, or *Research in Nursing*, by Holly Skodol Wilson, will be helpful not only in thinking about research but in writing about it. Wilson, for example, gives a general guide for writing a research proposal, detailed guidelines for writing a standard consent form (with an illustration), a checklist for writing a protocol for an institutional review board, suggestions for writing research questions, examples of hypotheses, and guidelines for presenting research in talks, articles, and books. While Polit and Hungler do not deal so directly with writing, they also offer a good deal of help, providing illustrations of research problem statements, suggestions for writing a literature review (with an example), guidelines for formulating hypotheses, with a long list of examples, detailed suggestions for constructing questionnaires and interview schedules, and a discussion of what a research report should contain.

A good statistics book is also an important reference. There's a nicely written introduction to the subject by Derek Rowntree, called *Statistics Without Tears: A Primer for Non-Mathematicians* (in paperback). The emphasis is not on calculations but on ideas; the book is designed to help one think statistically.

In addition to these basic books, it is helpful to have one or two general books on writing. The one I like best is William Zinsser's *On Writing Well: An Informal Guide to Writing Nonfiction*, in its third edition. Zinsser focuses not on technical or scientific writing but on more general types of essays, yet his advice is good for everyone and he follows it himself; the book is written clearly and with humanity and humor. Zinsser also has a book on *Writing with a Word Processor*, if you are interested in using that tool.

There are a few books on writing specifically for nurses, all in paperback. *Professional Writing for Nurses* by Philip C. Kolin and Janeen L. Kolin contains a basic guide to usage and discusses client care documentation, student writing, report writing, and professional writing. There is a chapter on writing an article and one on writing a book, though the focus is not on writing about research. *The Nurse's Writing Handbook* by Anita Gandolfo and Judy Romano reviews the basic rules of grammar and punctuation, and discusses the writing process in clinical, academic, and professional settings. There is one chapter on writing for publication, but again the focus is not on research.

Clinical Writing for Health Professionals by Alice Robinson and Lucille Notter gives guidelines for what an article reporting research, an abstract, and a research grant proposal should contain. Andrea O'Connor's *Writing for Nursing Publications* and Susan K. Mirin's *Nurse's Guide to Writing for Publication* give basic advice on writing and publishing an article, though the emphasis is not on a research article. O'Connor focuses on the writing process and Mirin emphasizes the publication process. Both books contain lengthy appendixes describing various aspects of nursing journals.

Author's Guide to Journals in Nursing and Related Fields, edited by Steven D. Warner and Kathryn D. Schweer, is a comprehensive list of journals and addresses, with information on types of articles sought, major content areas, review procedures, and time lags.

Finally, whatever other books on writing you buy, you should certainly own the *Publication Manual of the American Psychological Association* (third edition). This is extremely useful in setting up reference citations in the text and preparing the reference list at the end of your thesis, dissertation, or article. And it also contains a great deal of advice about writing, editorial style, tables and figures, and typing the parts of a manuscript. The other style manuals are also helpful, but this is the easiest to use.

References

American Psychological Association. (1983). *Publication manual* (3rd ed.). Washington, DC.

Aquilino, M. L., & Ely, J. (1985). Parents and the sexuality of preschool children. *Pediatric Nursing, 11,* 41-46.

Dissertation Abstracts International. A: The Humanities and Social Sciences; B: The Sciences and Engineering. (1969). Ann Arbor: University Microfilms International.

Dorman, E. A., & Dawe, C. W. (1984). *The brief English handbook.* Boston: Little, Brown.

Fuller, E. O. (1983). Preparing an abstract of a nursing study. *Nursing Research, 32,* 316-317.

Gandolfo, A., & Romano, J. (1984). *The nurse's writing handbook.* Norwalk, Conn: Appleton-Century-Crofts.

Guth, H. P. (1982). *New English handbook.* Belmont, CA: Wadsworth.

Johnson, E. D. (1982). *The handbook of good English.* New York: Facts on File Publications.

Jordan, J., & Meckler, J. R. (1982). The relationship between life change events, social supports, and dysmenorrhea. *Research in Nursing and Health, 5,* 73-79.

Kolin, P. C., & Kolin, J. L. (1980). *Professional writing for nurses in education, practice, and research.* St. Louis: C. V. Mosby.

Leggett, G., Mead, C. D., & Charvat, W. (1978). *Handbook for writers* (7th ed.). Englewood Cliffs, NJ: Prentice-Hall.

McCloskey, J. C., & Swanson, E. (1982). Publishing opportunities for nurses: A comparison of 100 journals. *Image: The Journal of Nursing Scholarship, 14,* 50-56.

McQueen, W. A. (1979). *A short guide to English composition* (3rd ed.). Belmont, CA: Wadsworth.

Mirin, S. K. (1981). *Nurse's guide to writing for publication.* Wakefield, MA: Nursing Resources.

O'Connor, A. B. (1976). *Writing for nursing publications.* Thorofare, NJ: Slack.

Polit, D. F., & Hungler, B. P. (1978). *Nursing research: Principles and methods.* Philadelphia: J.B. Lippincott.

Roberts, W. H. (1984). *The writer's companion: A short handbook.* Boston: Little, Brown.

Robinson, A. M., & Notter, L. E. (1982). *Clinical writing for health professionals*. Bowie, MD: Brady.

Rowntree, D. (1982). *Statistics without tears: A primer for non-mathematicians*. New York: Scribner.

Strunk, W., Jr., & White, E. B. (1979). *The elements of style* (3rd ed.). New York: Macmillan.

Sultz, H. A., & Sherwin, F. S. (1981). *Grant writing for health professionals*. Boston: Little, Brown.

Swanson, E., & McCloskey, J. C. (1982). The manuscript review process of nursing journals. *Image: The Journal of Nursing Scholarship, 14*, 72-76.

Warner, S. D., & Schweer, K. D. (Eds.). (1982). *Author's guide to journals in nursing and related fields*. New York: Haworth Press.

Wilson, H. S. (1985). *Research in nursing*. Menlo Park, CA: Addison-Wesley.

Zinsser, W. K. (1983). *Writing with a word processor*. New York: Harper & Row.

Zinsser, W. K. (1985). *On writing well: An informal guide to writing nonfiction* (3rd ed.). New York: Harper & Row.

Index

Related Titles of Interest

FROM PRACTICE TO GROUNDED THEORY: Qualitative Research in Nursing by W. Carole Chenitz, RN, EdD and Janice M. Swanson, RN, PhD

A pioneering guide to understanding, using, and applying grounded theory in qualitative nursing research.

#12960/304 pp/Paperbound/1986

RESEARCH IN NURSING by Holly Skodol Wilson, RN, PhD, FAAN

An AJN Book of the Year, written with style and authority, consistently modeling the relevance of nursing research to nursing practice and the profession.

#09737/575 pp/Hardbound/1985

FROM NOVICE TO EXPERT: Excellence and Practice in Nursing Education by Patricia Benner, RN, PhD

Winner of the 1984 AJN Book of the Year in Education and Research, and a testimonial to the importance of nursing. Includes many clear, colorful examples from actual nursing practice, presented in nurses' own words.

#00299/307 pp/Softbound/1984

To order, write Addison-Wesley, Jacob Way, Reading, MA 01867 or call 617-944-3700